A Resident's Guide to Psychiatric Education

CRITICAL ISSUES IN PSYCHIATRY
An Educational Series for Residents and Clinicians

Series Editor: Sherwyn M. Woods, M.D., Ph.D.
                   University of Southern California School of Medicine
                   Los Angeles, California

A RESIDENT'S GUIDE TO PSYCHIATRIC EDUCATION
Edited by Michael G. G. Thompson, M.D.

STATES OF MIND: Analysis of Change in Psychotherapy
Mardi J. Horowitz, M.D.

DRUG AND ALCOHOL ABUSE: A Clinical Guide to
     Diagnosis and Treatment
Mark A. Schuckit, M.D.

A Resident's Guide to Psychiatric Education

Edited by

Michael G. G. Thompson, M.D.

Director of Education
Department of Psychiatry
University of Western Ontario
and
Medical Director and Chief of Staff
London Psychiatric Hospital
London, Ontario, Canada

PLENUM MEDICAL BOOK COMPANY • New York and London

Library of Congress Cataloging in Publication Data

Main entry under title:

A Resident's guide to psychiatric education.

(Critical issues in psychiatry)
Bibliography: p.
Includes index.
1. Psychiatry — Handbooks, manuals, etc. 2. Psychiatry — Study and teach-
ing (Residency) I. Thompson, Michael G. G. II. Series. [DNLM: 1. Psychiatry —
Education. WM18 R433]
RC454.4.R47   616.8'9   78-15961
ISBN-13: 978-1-4615-8197-0   e-ISBN-13: 978-1-4615-8195-6
DOI: 10.1007/978-1-4615-8195-6

© 1979 Plenum Publishing Corporation
227 West 17th Street, New York, N.Y. 10011

Plenum Medical Book Company is an imprint of Plenum Publishing Corporation

Foreword

This is the inaugural volume of the new series: *Critical Issues in Psychiatry: An Educational Series for Residents and Clinicians*. It is an appropriate beginning, for this book represents a milestone in the evolution of psychiatric education. For the first time, there will now be a single place where one can find a comprehensive collection of educational goals and objectives to define the broad spectrum of knowledge and skills essential for general and child psychiatry. This collection does not represent the bias of a single educator or program. Rather, it consists of a consensually validated ranking of relative importance for each educational goal and objective as determined by a large and international sampling of experienced psychiatric educators, as well as an editorial board with some of the most distinguished names in psychiatric education. It is even possible to tell at a glance whether the ranked level of importance is the same or different within several national groups, for example Canadians vs. Americans.

This book is intended for all students of psychiatry. It is particularly valuable to residents in training, but equally so for experienced clinicians preparing for Board examination or simply attending to the process of continuing education and intellectual renewal. While it might well be used by an institution to delineate the dimensions of a training program in psychiatry, it is intended primarily for the self-evaluation and self-monitoring of one's growth as a psychiatrist. The knowledge base in our field is growing exponentially. This has accentuated the need for a comprehensive instrument to first evaluate areas of strength and weakness across the dimensions of modern psychiatry, and then to direct study and experience. This is obviously most useful when it can be done in terms of educational objectives which are relevant to generally agreed upon standards of knowledge and skills. By noting the attainment of each item, the resident or clinician is able to record and follow his or her growth during the period of formal training and on into professional life.

The log book can be used similarly to record clinical experiences with patients across many dimensions: diagnosis, age, sex, social class, etc. It also serves to record experience and the development of skills in a wide variety of clinical activities: diagnostic interviews and procedures, somatic and pharmacologic intervention, behavioral therapies, marital and family therapies, group therapies, individual psychotherapies, etc. This is of particular importance to the trainee who must take care that his or her education is not skewed too heavily in one direction (type of patient, diagnosis, modality of treatment), or, of even more serious concern, lacking with regard to some important aspect of clinical skill development or experience.

The reference material, the listing of psychiatric publications, the names and addresses of psychiatric organizations, and the other useful information all contribute toward the goal of providing a complete resource book for the education of the psychiatrist. To inaugurate this series we have conspired to produce a volume which might well be regarded as an educational essential for anyone about to become, in the process of becoming, or wishing to remain an excellent, knowledgeable, and modern clinical psychiatrist. We hope its usefulness to you, the reader and student, will prove the attainment of that goal.

Sherwyn M. Woods, M.D., Ph.D.
Series Editor

Preface

The contents of this guide are an attempt to offer to the psychiatric resident some guidelines in the broad field of psychiatry.

The guide is not meant to be static or completely comprehensive. It should be subject to continuing revision through feedback by residents, faculty, and other interested persons. It is hoped that the gradual evolution of such a guide will lead to more precision in the setting of educational objectives and more objectivity in the evaluation of the attainment of such objectives. Because it delineates "objectives" and not "content," it will not require revision either as frequently or as extensively as a comparable textbook.

This volume is not a guide to the examinations, nor is it a blueprint for what should be taught in any one department or asked at the examinations. It should in no way be interpreted as a document that delineates the field precisely.

The effort of compiling this guide was a collaborative one. While acknowledging the indispensable contributions of many others, with special appreciation to those mentioned in the various acknowledgments, and to the editorial board, the editor takes responsibility for the final format with any omissions or inconsistencies it may contain.

Special thanks are given for secretarial assistance in the preparation of this manuscript to Lois Bolger and Peggy Coleman, London Psychiatric Hospital, London, Ontario; Fran Eggleston, University Hospital, London, Ontario; and Mary Lou DeMarco, Toronto, Ontario.

Finally, a *very special thanks* to the scores of psychiatrists whose names are not listed here but who contributed many hours critically reviewing this work and whose suggestions have been incorporated herein.

Michael G. G. Thompson, M.D.

Editor's Introduction

This manual for residents is both a guide to and a means of monitoring one's educational development in psychiatry. Specifically, the prime purpose of this book is to outline that which the resident should be able to do in order to show that he or she has attained a sufficient level of knowledge and skill to practice as a specialist in general psychiatry. The central core of the manual is therefore Chapter 1, Terminal and Enabling Objectives.

The following short sections, which directly relate to and complement this core, have also been included: a list of recommended training experiences to assist the resident in the application of knowledge and the acquisition of new clinical skills (Chapter 2); a means of evaluating one's own training center from the point of view of assessing its ability to meet one's didactic and experiential needs (Chapter 3); a chapter on "extra" objectives for training in the subspecialty area of child psychiatry (Chapter 4); and, last, Appendices A–D, which comprise a listing of professional associations, a brief guide to the psychiatric literature, official statements as to the essentials of residency training in psychiatry, and an introductory reading list for Chapter 1.

The driving force behind this guide has been the continual insistence on the part of residents for the profession to establish more clearly the parameters of our field. It has been compiled in the belief that although we as psychiatrists must learn to live with ambiguity, the delineation of our area of expertise does not have to be ambiguous.

Michael G. G. Thompson, M.D.

Contents

Chapter 2
Recommended Training Experiences and Skills: A Log Book

Appendix A
Professional Associations

Appendix B
A Guide to the Psychiatric Literature

Appendix C
Training Requirements

Appendix D
Introductory Reading List for Chapter 1

Chapter 1

Terminal and Enabling Objectives

Editor's Introduction

Each university department of psychiatry has its own unique cadre of specialists, teaching centers, and central themes at any given time. The core common to all the teaching programs consists of a basic minimum number of areas that a graduate psychiatrist must have both knowledge of and skill in. Which areas, what knowledge, and what skills—these are the perplexing and overtly unanswered questions. Skill is both inherent and taught. The portion that can be taught is necessary, but not sufficient. The "inherent" component, however, introduces the whole problem of "who" should be permitted to train in psychiatry, and it will not be dealt with in this training guide. Similarly, the "hows," "whens," and "wheres" of process and technique in the training programs will be omitted. This chapter deals only with the question of "what" in terms of statements, i.e., enabling objectives, as to what the postgraduate student must be able to do to show that the necessary minimum core knowledge and skill to be a psychiatrist have been attained.

The work on precise delineation of goals and objectives was initiated in the fall of 1973 by the members of Coordinators of Psychiatric Education (C.O.P.E.). The membership of this organization consists of directors of postgraduate training in psychiatry at each of the medical schools across Canada. Each director was asked to set out, in collaboration with the staff and postgraduate students of his center, a list of enabling objectives delineating the basic minimum that a psychiatrist must be able to do to show that he or she has attained the required level of knowledge and skill in a given area of learning. That which could be reasonably subsumed under the broad rubric of psychiatry had been rather arbitrarily divided into twenty sections, and each center was assigned at least one section as its topic area. Each center's contribution was then reviewed by another center. This process was repeated two or more times for most sections before the final submissions were made. These sections were then revised and edited by the editor, and the titles of the various university contributions became the basis for the table of contents.

Concurrently and independently, the American Association of Directors of Psychiatric Residency Training (AADPRT) had set up a task force on curriculum. Both groups, virtually without knowledge of each other's work, were wrestling with precisely the same problem: how to delineate more precisely for the resident that which he must be able to know and do. When communication finally occurred, the AADPRT's task force made the decision to take the C.O.P.E. manuscript as a baseline. A very thorough method for critically reviewing and assigning each objective a priority was initiated by this group and subsequently carried out by selected directors of residency training programs, chairmen of university psychiatric departments, national board examiners, and examiners of the Royal Colleges and psychiatrists in general psychiatric practice from Australia, Canada, Great Britain, and the United States.

These psychiatrists were asked either to assign each objective one of the following numerical ratings:

1. Required of all residents (high emphasis)
2. Moderate emphasis
3. Touched upon or optional

or to suggest that the objective be changed or deleted.* A mean score based on these ratings was calculated for each of the more than 800 objectives; this score could range from 1.00 to 3.00. A mean score of 1.00 would indicate that everyone had rated that objective as essential for all residents. A mean score of 3.00 would indicate that all the respondents had rated that objective as "Touched upon or optional." The following cutoff points for a ①–④ rating system were established:†

① for means from 1.00 to 1.10 inclusive
The objective was rated essential for all residents by 90% of the respondents. This category comprises 20% of the objectives.

② for means from 1.11 to 1.37 inclusive
The objective was rated essential for all residents by more than approximately 75–80% of the respondents. This category comprises 28% of the objectives.

Thus, categories ① and ② together account for 48% of the objectives.

③ for means from 1.38 to 1.99 inclusive
For the most part, respondents felt that an objective so rated should be given at least moderate emphasis by the resident. This category comprises 37% of the objectives.

---

*A fourth rating, "delete," was thus available but was virtually never used by the respondents.
†The percentages of objectives in the four categories reflect data gleaned from responses to Sections I–XVIII and XX. Ratings for Section XIX, Gender and Psychiatry, were obtained by a later questionnaire.

④ for means from 2.00 to 3.00 inclusive
Responses in this category indicate questionnaire ratings ranging from moderate emphasis to touched upon or optional. This category comprises 15% of the objectives.

In addition the responses were grouped according to nationality and were statistically analyzed in order to determine if significant differences existed between the responses from Australia (n = 12),* Canada (n = 20), and the United States (n = 20). Wherever the difference reached a level of significance of .005 or better, the priority rating allocated by each national group has been indicated in addition to the overall priority rating to the left of the objective in the following manner:

②▽①△   1. To be able to . . .

where:

② is an overall priority ranking of 2
▽ is an Australian ranking of 2
① is a Canadian ranking of 1
△ is an American ranking of 3

Whenever the differences between the national groups reached a level between .005 and .01 this has been noted in a footnote. Whenever, in a group of objectives, a definite trend is apparent but a significance level of .01 is not reached, this trend is also noted by a footnote.

Due to comments made during this extensive in-depth prepublication review, some objectives were significantly altered and a number of new ones were added. The new objectives are considered important by the editor, but were not subjected to review by questionnaire and are therefore not given ratings.

The manuscript was then reviewed and revised with the assistance of the editorial board prior to publication.

The content of each section represents a "comprehensive core." The postgraduate must know something about every major area and topic, but to allow for individual differences, which will always exist, slightly more is included in each section than is considered absolutely essential by all the training centers.

Although the majority of practicing psychiatrists could not at any given moment recall enough information to meet all the objectives outlined herein, it is still a maxim that once a thorough attempt to master the whole subject area has been made, it becomes a relatively simple task to retrieve and understand previously learned basic principles and concepts, integrate them with newer advances in the field, and utilize this knowledge in one's practice at times when it is important to do so.

In delineating the "what" of psychiatry, those involved hope that most of the core objectives are "universal" in the sense of both time and content.

*Each Australian questionnaire was filled out by a group of psychiatrists at a different center.

This chapter is *not* a textbook; rather, it is an outline in the form of enabling objectives of core material in psychiatry.

This chapter deals with three identified problems:

1. The need for a clear outline delineating subject areas for psychiatric residents.
2. The need for uniform definition of what is an acceptable basic minimum level of knowledge and skill in each area.
3. The need for an orienting or organizing thread or theme (Fig. 1).

In the editing process, although the majority of the "objectives" suggested by the various centers are included, the editor has taken the liberty of altering both the format and the content of many of these submissions to minimize redundancy and standardize the format.

The format is as follows:

The upper case Roman numerals I through XX designate the twenty major sections into which this chapter is divided.

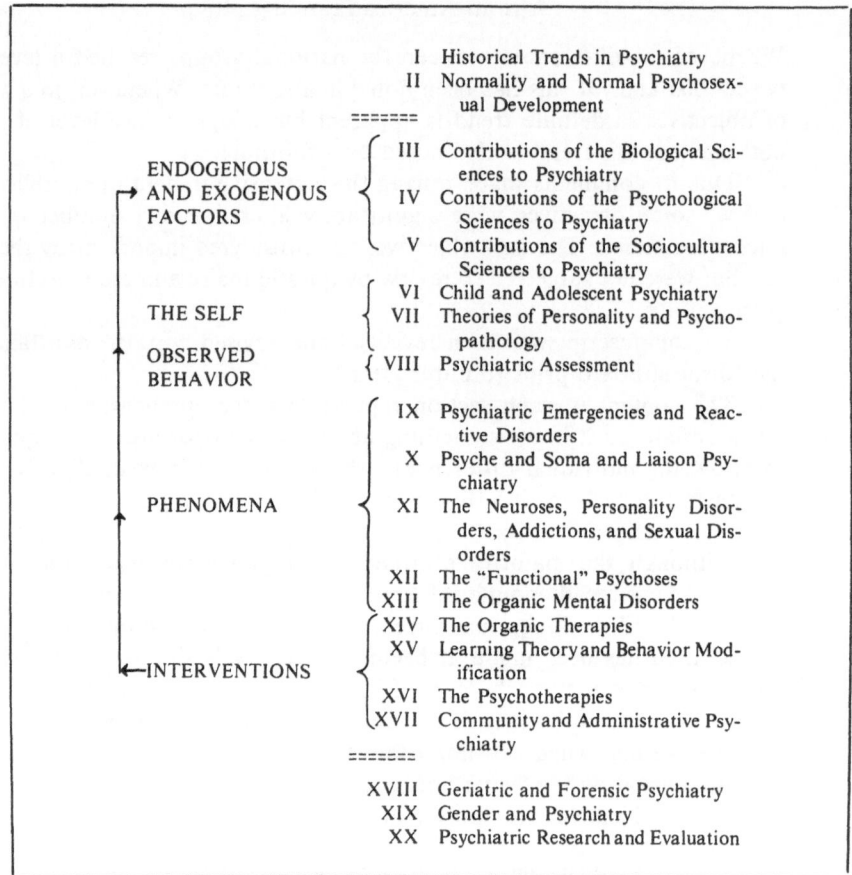

Fig. 1. A "systems" method for ordering sections.

Upper case letters A, B, C, etc., designate the topics (if any) into which a section is divided.

Lower case Roman numerals i, ii, iii, etc., designate the subtopics (if any) into which a topic is divided.

The subdivisions (if any) of each section are listed under the heading GENERAL PLAN.

For a given section, topic, or subtopic, as appropriate, there is a statement of one or more TERMINAL OBJECTIVES.

Under each subdivision is a list of ENABLING OBJECTIVES, plus more specific content-oriented "guides." Arabic numbers 1, 2, 3, etc., designate these enabling objectives; subdivisions are designated by 1.1, 1.2, 1.3, etc., and further subdivisions, where necessary, by 1.1.1, 1.1.2, 1.1.3, etc. Lower case letters a, b, c, etc., designate aspects of a given enabling objective (or subdivision thereof) to which attention should be given.

Six further statements concerning the style in which this document is written deserve attention:

First, all lists are open-ended, and it is hoped that as further objectives are added and old ones deleted or modified, the teaching centers will communicate these changes to the editor.

Second, the "guides," being content-oriented, will constantly be modified by those using the manual.

Third, to keep the text to a reasonable length, the enabling objectives are of a different order of specificity than true "behavioral objectives" in that more than one point is made in each. It should also be noted at this juncture that some of the guides include lists of authors' names. The purpose of this listing was not to force the student to learn the work of a particular author, at times a futile exercise, but rather to give an introduction to the literature in that particular area. If such lists are used in this way, they become aids to learning, rather than onerous tasks.

Fourth, it will also be noted by the reader that there are marked differences in the detail in which the areas are covered. The reason is that some of the areas are covered in other sections of the guide; for example, the neuroses in child psychiatry (Section VI.A.ii, objectives 1 and 2) would have many of the same objectives as the general section on the neuroses (Section XI.A) in the manual.

Fifth, the suggested introductory reading list (Appendix D) is intended only as an initial guide. The "major" references are meant to be fairly well rounded, general introductions to the content material required to meet the objectives in a particular section, while the "other" references are meant as initial reading in specific subtopic areas.

Last, concerning the categorization of mental disorders, in the early drafts of this guide, both the ICDA-8 and the DSM II were used for Sections IX–XIII. Recently, terms from DSM III were added. In revising for publication, the editor has therefore attempted to increase both internal consistency and clarity by substituting and adding phrases that are for the

most part self-explanatory or descriptive. The overriding principles have
been clarity and universality of objectives. Thus, in Sections XI and XII, although the DSM III categories were more specific, the groupings of categories for purposes of writing objectives were more usefully left in broad general areas that corresponded to the neuroses and personality disorders for
Section XI and the functional psychoses for Section XII as per the ICDA and
the DSM II classification schemes. For the purposes of this guide, the controversy surrounding whether or not the affective disorders should be together or placed in two sections (psychotic vs. nonpsychotic) and whether
or not simple and latent schizophrenia (and borderline states) should be
left with the functional psychoses (ICDA) or placed with the personality
disorders (DSM III) was considered from the point of view of the appropriateness of the objectives to the topic in question. The editor's decision
was again to leave the divisions as they are found in the ICD and DSM II
classification schemes for these two sections of the manual, noting where
appropriate the relevant DSM III categories and positioning thereof.

In conclusion, the editor, on behalf of the contributors, would like to
emphasize again that the production of this guide represents an ongoing
collaborative effort and that in no way is the guide meant to be a static
statement.

Section I.   Historical Trends in Psychiatry

TERMINAL OBJECTIVE

To understand the significance of the history of psychiatry for modern
clinical practice and research.

ENABLING OBJECTIVES

④   *1. Be able to give a short summary of the contributions to modern psy-
    chiatry of historical, religious, and medical discourses on the subject
    of the body and the spirit.*

    Guide: Include discourses from the following eras:
    1.1. Greek society
    1.2. Roman Empire
    1.3. Middle Ages
    1.4. Renaissance and 17th century
    1.5. Judeo-Christian
    1.6. . . .
    1.7. . . .

④   *2. Be able to discuss briefly the historical development of the moral treat-
    ment of the insane (18th and 19th centuries).*

    Guide: Include contributions made by workers in the following countries:
    2.1. Italy
    2.2   England

2.3. France
2.4. United States
2.5. . . .
2.6. . . .

③ 3. *Be able to state the origins of the classifications of mental illnesses (19th century and beginning of the 20th century).*

Guide: Note in particular the contributions made by physicians in the following countries:
3.1. France
3.2. England
3.3. Germany
3.4. United States
3.5. . . .
3.6. . . .

③ 4. *Be able to discuss the major trends in contemporary psychiatry.*

Guide: Include:
4.1. Birth of dynamic psychiatry
    4.1.1. Pre-Freudian
    4.1.2. Freud
    4.1.3. The dissidents—Jung. Adler, other interpersonal theorists
    4.1.4. Ego psychologists
    4.1.5. M. Klein *et al.*
    4.1.6. . . .
    4.1.7. . . .
4.2. Progress of biological psychiatry
    4.2.1. Contributions of neurology at the turn of the century
    4.2.2. Biological treatments
        a. Malaria therapy
        b. Insulin and ECT
        c. Psychosurgery
        d. Psychopharmacology
    4.2.3. . . .
    4.2.4. . . .
4.3. Beginnings of psychosomatic medicine
4.4. Contributions of child psychiatry
4.5. Origins of community psychiatry
4.6. Antipsychiatry movement
4.7. Contributions of psychophysiology and experimental psychology—behavior therapy
4.8. . . .
4.9. . . .

④ 5. *Be able to outline the historical origins of the mind–body dichotomy.*

④ 6. *Be able to show the changes in the attitude of society toward mental illnesses over time.*

Note: Objectives 5 and 6 may be considered as "guides" to objectives 1–4.

③ 7. *Be able to state briefly the contributions to psychiatry of well-known authors in medicine and the social sciences.*

Guide: Be able to state for each author:

a. Area of special expertise.

b. Period in which the author worked

c. Basic tenets of the author's theoretical position

d. Fundamental contributions to modern psychiatric practice

8. . . .

9. . . .

Section II.   Normality and Normal Psychosexual Development

GENERAL PLAN

A. Concept of Normality

B. Normal Psychosexual Development

A. Concept of Normality

TERMINAL OBJECTIVE

To be able to understand the importance of the concept of "normality" in psychiatry.

ENABLING OBJECTIVES

② 1. *Be able to discuss the concept of "normality."*

   Guide: Include the following areas:

   1.1. Dimensions (normality as health, ideal, average, and normality as a relative concept)

   1.2. Relationship to age

   1.3. Adaptive patterns to stress

   1.4. Society and culture and "change" with time

   1.5. Cross-cultural "universals"

   1.6. Role of the psychiatrist in defining normality

   1.7. Importance of the concept in research

   1.8. Influence on North American concepts of normality of Judeo-Christian ideals, materialism, and individualisn

   1.9. . . .

   1.10. . . .

2. *With reference to clinical material, be able to critically assess "normality" and deviance from "normality" both for the patient and for the patient in relation to the examiner.*

   Guide: Note in particular the following factors:

   a. Age

   b. Society and culture (tolerance of the social group)

    c. Legal responsibility

    d. Type and immediacy of stress

    e. Biological (puberty, menopause, individual differences in response pattern)

    f. . . .

    g. . . .

3. *With reference to normal families, be able to state the effects of each of the following events on each of the family members:*

    3.1. Birth of a sibling (effect of temperament on family members)

    3.2. Illness of a family member

    3.3. Beginning or changing school

    3.4. Vacation

    3.5. Change of residence

    3.6. Change of breadwinner's employment

    3.7. Death of a family member or close relative

    3.8. . . .

    3.9. . . .

4. . . .

5. . . .

B. Normal Psychosexual Development

TERMINAL OBJECTIVE

To know the psychological and physiological aspects of normal sexual behavior and its development through different phases of life from infancy to maturity and old age.

ENABLING OBJECTIVES

③   *1. Be able to outline briefly major contributions to our understanding of normal psychosexual development and sexual functioning.*

    Guide: Include:

    1.1. Psychological aspects

        a. Helene Duetsch

        b. Erik Erickson

        c. Sigmund Freud

        d. Karl Jung

        e. Melanie Klein

        f. . . .

        g. . . .

    1.2. Descriptive and physiological aspects

        a. Masters and Johnson

        b. Money, J., Hampson, J. G., and Kinsey, J. L.

        c. Pomeroy and Martin

        d. . . .

        e. . . .

     1.3. . . .

     1.4. . . .

②   *2. Be able to outline briefly the importance of psychosexual factors to clinical psychiatry.*

     Guide: Include:

     2.1. Sexual identity

     2.2. Gender identity (special attention to recent literature)

     2.3. Gender role

     2.4. . . .

     2.5. . . .

③   *3. Be able to state the effect of physical disabilities, illnesses, and medications on sexual desire and behavior.*

    4. Be able to compare and contrast the male and female life cycles, with emphasis on the dilemmas associated with achievement, motivation, affiliation, sexuality, femininity, and masculinity.

     Guide: Include the following areas:

     4.1. Socialization of children, adolescents, and adults

     4.2. Pregnancy, childbirth, and the puerperium

     4.3. The middle years and the menopause

     4.4. Old age

     4.5. . . .

     4.6. . . .

  5. . . .

  6. . . .

Note: Objectives for many factors that relate directly to normal psychosexual functioning have been placed in Section VII.A, Personality Development and the Life Cycle, and Section XIX, Gender and Psychiatry.

Section III. Contributions of the Biological Sciences to Psychiatry

Introduction: Changes in the Delivery of Mental Health Care

One of the consequences of community psychiatry has been the recognition that qualified nonmedical professionals can manage many aspects of psychosocial distress that had previously been regarded as the exclusive responsibility of psychiatrists. This change will allow psychiatrists to devote themselves with greater vigor to those clinical problems that call for biomedical knowledge; the need to keep abreast of advances in biological science is likely to become more urgent than ever.

    During the last fifty years, psychiatry was identified in some quarters wholly with the practice of psychotherapy, especially in the influential academic centers of the United States. An unfortunate outcome of this identification was the extrusion from the psychiatric territory of any disorder that became treatable by physical means or seemed otherwise "too medical," e.g., CNS syphilis, some forms of mental retardation, delirium tremens. (Indeed, the treatment of recurrent affective disorders with lithium is even now regarded as a fitting business for internists rather than psychiatrists in at least one urban region.) This trend will probably become completely reversed in the near future, and clinical problems that depend for their solution on biomedical knowledge will be viewed as the very paradigms of psychiatric activity. With this probability in mind, more detail has been retained in this section on the biological sciences than in many other sections of this chapter.

GENERAL PLAN

A. Core Knowledge in Neuropsychiatry
B. Core Knowledge in Neuroendocrinology
C. Core Knowledge in Neurochemistry and Neurophysiology and the relationship of These Sciences to Psychiatric Disorders
D. Memory
E. Sleep and Dreams
F. Experimental Psychopathology
    i. Psychomimetic Agents (Euphorohallucinogens)
    ii. Experimental Neurosis
    iii. Sensory Deprivation
    iv. Sleep Deprivation
G. Specialized Tests in Neurological Investigation
H. Neurological Correlates of Specialized Procedures

TERMINAL OBJECTIVE

To gain an understanding of the basic genetic, neurophysiological, and neurochemical mechanisms underlying behavior.

A. Core Knowledge in Neuropsychiatry

ENABLING OBJECTIVES

1. Be able to demonstrate a working knowledge of basic neurological signs and syndromes, including:

③   *1.1. The symptomatology, neurophysiology, and neuropathology of spastic and flaccid paresis, the akinetic–hypertonic extrapyramidal syndrome, and the various types of extrapyramidal hyperkinesis, the different types of epileptic seizures, their respective localizations, and their EEG manifestations.*

③   *1.2. The different qualitative types of hypesthesias, their distribution according to the different localization of the lesion (peripheral, spinal, cerebral), and the pathways of their conduction. Of particular importance is the basic knowledge of the visual pathways from the retina to the calcarine region, the various types of hemianopia, and other forms of visual field defects and their localization. The same applies to the acoustic, olfactory, and gustatory pathways, although less need be known in these areas.*

③   *1.3. The various forms of ataxia (peripheral, spinal, cerebellar, frontal) and their combination with other neurological signs, e.g., ophthalmoplegia in Wernicke's disease and other mesencephalic lesions.*

1.4. . . .

1.5. . . .

2. *Be able to demonstrate a working knowledge of the general principles of brain functioning and their physiological and pathophysiological expressions:*

③   *2.1. The reticuloactivating system and the nonspecific corticopetal projections. Arousal, level of consciousness, from normal awareness to clouded states and coma. Physiology and pathology of sleep.*

②   *2.2. The limbic system and the neurophysiology of the emotions—aggression, anxiety, depression, euphoria. The physiology and pathology of amygdala.*

②   *2.3. The hippocampus–fornix–mammillary body–thalamus–cingulum system and its pathology. The amnestic syndrome, short- and long-term memory.*

③   *2.4. The gnosopractic (neocortical) functions and their pathology. This would include the various forms of aphasia, alexia, agraphia, agnosia, and apraxia, the Gerstmann syndrome, autotopagnosia and anosognosia and their relationship to handedness.*

②   *2.5. The endocrine–autonomic nervous system–hypothalamus functions and their pathology. This would include drinking, eating, temperature regulation, sexual activity, and preparation for fight and flight.*

②   *2.6. The functions of the different lobes—frontal, temporal, parietal, and occipital—and their participation in perception, cognition, and motivation.*

2.7. . . .

2.8. . . .

3. *. . .*

4. *. . .*

B. Core Knowledge in Neuroendocrinology

ENABLING OBJECTIVES

③   *1. Be able to list and briefly discuss hormones and the endocrine glands that produce them.*

Guide: The following should be included:

1.1.   Neurosecretions—vasopressin, oxytocin

1.2.   Thyroid control—TRH, TSH plus thyroid hormone T_3, T_4

1.3.   Adrenal control—CRF, ACTH plus adrenal hormones

    1.4.   Control of gonadotropins, LH by LRH and dopamine

    1.5.   Control of follicle-stimulating hormone (FSH) by FRH and dopamine

    1.6.   Control of GH by somatostatin (GH release inhibiting factor) and by GRF

    1.7.   Control of prolactin by prolactin inhibiting factor (PIF) and L-dopa

    1.8.   Pineal melatonin

    1.9.   Melanocyte-stimulating hormone inhibiting factor (MIF)

    1.10. . . .

    1.11. . . .

③   2. *Be able to discuss briefly, using the principles of general systems theory, the interaction and feedback control mechanisms of the various elements of the neuroendocrine system.*

    Guide: Hypothalamic–pituitary system

③   3. *Be able to state the present state of scientific knowledge concerning the relevance of neuroendocrinology to psychiatric symptomatology.*

    Guide: This could include such topics as:

    3.1. The psychoses

    3.2. Psychosomatic disorders

    3.3. Other "postulated" relationships, including:

        3.3.1.   Testosterone and aggression

        3.3.2.   GH and LH to anorexia

        3.3.3.   Androgens (prenatal) and sex orientation

        3.3.4.   LH and FSH and psychogenic amenorrhea

        3.3.5.   FSH, LH, prolactin, and pseudocyesis

        3.3.6.   Testosterone and homosexuality

        3.3.7.   GH plus environment and psychosocial dwarfism

        3.3.8.   ACTH, adrenal steroids, and depression and euphoria

        3.3.9.   LRH and mating behavior

        3.3.10. Somatostatin and calming and other behavioral effects

        3.3.11. The relationship between activity restraint, acute danger (stress), withdrawal and/or depression, hypoglycemia, sexual stimulation, and CS, GH, prolactin, and the limbic system

        3.3.12. . . .

        3.3.13. . . .

State in each case above:

a. *what is known concerning the mechanisms of the suggested relationship*

b. *The neurotransmitter controls for each*

c. *The clinical picture*

d. *Implications for preventions: primary, secondary, and tertiary*

3.4. . . .

3.5. . . .

③   *4. Be able to demonstrate an integrated knowledge concerning the bio-
      logical concomitants of the stress reaction.*

     Guide: The following factors should be considered:
     4.1. Limbic system, the hypothalamus, the pituitary and adrenal glands
     4.2. The hippocampus, median forebrain bundle, septum, and amygdaloid
     4.3. Norepinephrine and serotonin
     4.4. . . .
     4.5. . . .

③   *5. Be able to relate for objectives 1–4 the possible significance for liaison
      psychiatry of recent findings in neuroendocrinology.*

     Guide: Include:
     5.1. The patterns of GH and cortisol response to cardiac catheterization
     5.2. . . .
     5.3. . . .

    6. . . .
    7. . . .

C. Core Knowledge in Neurochemistry and Neurophysiology and the Relationship of These Sciences to Psychiatric Disorders

ENABLING OBJECTIVES

③   *1. Be able to describe the structure and function of the synapse.*

     Guide: Include:
     1.1. Anatomical structure (including subcellular organelles and struc-
         ture of the neuron)
     1.2. Structure of the membranes
     1.3. Neurotransmitters
     1.4. Metabolic processes during transmission, e.g., for neurotrans-
         mitters, their synthesis, storage, release, action, and breakdown
     1.5. Electrolyte changes during impulse transmission
     1.6. Pre- and postsynaptic inhibition
     1.7. Application of the principles of general systems theory to electro-
         chemical events in impulse transmission (very briefly)
     1.8. . . .
     1.9. . . .

②   *2. Be able to discuss the distribution and metabolism of the neutotrans-
      mitters and their functional relevance to psychiatry.*

     Guide: Include the distribution, biosynthesis, storage, release and up-
     take of:
     2.1. Norepinephrine
     2.2. Serotonin
     2.3. Dopamine (D and L)
     2.4. Methylated indoleamines

2.5. Gamma amino butyric acid

2.6. Tyramine

2.7. . . .

2.8. . . .

Where appropriate, use examples in the discussion such as depression, schizophrenia, Gilles de la Tourette, parkinsonism, and arousal.

③   3. *Be able to discuss briefly electrolyte and water balance and its relevance to psychiatric disorders.*

      Guide: Include manic–depressive psychosis.

④   4. *Be able to discuss briefly protein metabolism and its relevance to psychiatric disorders.*

      Guide: Include alpha-2 globulin, antibodies (Heath), etc.

②   5. *Be able to state what is known at present about the neurochemical response of the central nervous system to the "biological" therapies.*

      Guide: Pay particular attention to the response of neurotransmitters synthesis, storage, action, and breakdown— to:

      5.1. Psychopharmacological agents

      5.2. ECT

      5.3. Reserpine

      5.4. . . .

      5.5. . . .

②   6. *Be able to list and discuss briefly the current biochemical theories of the affective disorders, the schizophrenic group of illnesses, and the anxiety states, noting in particular information referred to in objectives 1–5 above.*

③   7. *Be able to discuss basic research strategies in psychiatry and potential sources of error therein.*

④   8. *Be able to discuss briefly "balance" in neuropsychiatric disorders.*

      Guide: Make special reference to the ergotropic and trophotropic systems and include:

      a. The neurophysiological mechanisms involved

      b. Relationship to therapy, e.g., abreaction, ECT, behavior therapy, tranquilizers and antidepressants

      c. Relationship to illness— psychosomatic, neurotic, psychotic.

③   9. *Be able to discuss briefly biological rhythms, biological clocks, and the process of "switching" in psychiatric disorders.*

      Guide: Make special reference to:

      a. Manic–depressive psychosis

      b. Periodic catatonia

      c. Schizophrenia

      d. Other (such as migraine)

②   10. *Be able to outline the present state of scientific knowledge of the genetic transmission of psychiatric syndromes and predisposition to these syndromes.*

③   *11. In accomplishing objectives 1–10, the resident should refer briefly to the work of a few major investigators.*

        Guide:
        Kety (transmethylation)
        Himwich (dualistic theory involving catecholamines and indolamines)
        Friedhoff and Van Winke (DMPE)
        Osmond and Smythies (faulty noradrenalin metabolism)
        Heath (taraxein)
        Hoffer
        Coppen (sodium metabolism, serotonin, and depression)
        Schou (lithium)
        Schildkaut (catecholamine hypothesis)
        Hornykiewitz (dopamine)
        Axelrod
        Bergen *or* Frohman *or* Louzousky (alpha-2 globulin)
        Hess (trophotropic and ergotropic systems)
        Dement (sleep and dreams)
        Bunney (manic–depressive, switching)
        Gjessing (periodic catatonia)
        Kallmann (twins)
        Heston (twins)
        Slater (inheritance)
        Tienari (twins)
        Kety and Rosenthal (twins)
        Gottesman and Shields
        Carlsson, A. (catecholamine kinetics, dopaminergic kinetics)

12. . . .

13. . . .

D. Memory

ENABLING OBJECTIVES

③   *1. Be able to make pertinent statements about the present state of scientific knowledge of memory (immediate and short- and long-term), the process of storage, and the site thereof.*

        Guide: This knowledge should include such topics as:
        1.1. Type of memory
            1.1.1. "Immediate" memory (e.g., linguistic, pictorial, spontaneous decay)
            1.1.2. "Short-term" memory (e.g., units of information; interference; retention curves; effect of cooling, incising cortex, shock)
            1.1.3. "Long-term" memory
            1.1.4. . . .
            1.1.5. . . .

    1.2. Process of memory storage. including:

        1.2.1. "Registration" – including statements on the amnesias with notes on their:

            a. onset sudden or subacute

            b. recovery—complete or incomplete

            c. causation—the pathological processes, noting in particular the Wernicke–Korsakoff syndrome and the dementias

        1.2.2. "Retention"—including, e.g.. "Penfield's" bilateral hippocampal ablation, Korsakoff's

        1.2.3. "Recall"—including, e.g., repression, dissociative phenomena such as the fugue state, the paramnesias. hyperamnesia

        1.2.4. . . .

        1.2.5. . . .

    1.3. Site of storage:

        1.3.1. Lashley's "law" of mass action

        1.3.2. "Law" of equipotentiality

        1.3.3. Variation of effects of local lesions as a function of time

        1.3.4. Findings from "ablation" techniques

        1.3.5. Findings from electrophysiological techniques

        1.3.6. Findings from biochemical techniques

        1.3.7. Findings from split brain techniques

        1.3.8. . . .

        1.3.9. . . .

②   2. *Be able to list (and apply clinically) critical factors in the differential diagnosis of organically vs. psychologically caused amnesia.*

③   3. *Be able to state the effects of pharmacological agents on memory.*

    4. . . .

    5. . . .

E. Sleep and Dreams*

ENABLING OBJECTIVES

③   1. *Be able to describe the stages of sleep (NREM and REM).*

    Guide: Include statements on:

    1.1. Electrophysiology (EEG)

    1.2. Body activity (e.g.. muscle, respiratory. cardiovascular, temperature)

    1.3. Diurnal rhythm

    1.4. Dreaming

    1.5. Neuroanatomical and physiological mechanisms

    1.6. Neurochemical mechanisms

    1.7. Effects of sleep deprivation (physiological and behavioral)

---

*Although not reaching significance at the .01 level, Canadians rated each of the objectives on sleep one priority level above that which is indicated here.

1.8. . . .

1.9. . . .

Ⓖ *2. Be able to diagnose and describe the clinical picture, neurophysiological correlates, postulated etiology, and suitable treatment for disorders of sleep.*

Guide: Include:

2.1. "Excessive" sleep

    2.1.1. Sleep attacks

    2.1.2. Persistent sleepiness (simple hypersomnia)

    2.1.3. Hypersomnia with periodic respiration: Pickwickian syndrome, pure, Ondine's, mixed

    2.1.4. Hypersomnia with megaphagia (Klein–Levin syndrome)

    2.1.5. . . .

    2.1.6. . . .

2.2. "Inadequate" sleep

    2.2.1. Insomnia—causation: psychiatric, general medical, neurological

    2.2.2. Pseudoinsomnia

    2.2.3. . . .

    2.2.4. . . .

2.3. Psychosensory

    2.3.1. Hypnagogic hallucinations (excessive)

    2.3.2. Terrifying dreams

    2.3.3. Sleep terrors

    2.3.4. Sleep drunkenness (postdormital confusion)

    2.3.5. Peduncular hallucinosis

    2.3.6. . . .

    2.3.7. . . .

2.4. Motor

    2.4.1. Cataplexy

    2.4.2. Sleep paralysis

    2.4.3. Restless legs

    2.4.4. Jactatio capitis nocturna

    2.4.5. Somnambulism

    2.4.6. Somniloquy

    2.4.7. Snoring, etc.

    2.4.8. Bruxism

    2.4.9. . . .

    2.4.10. . . .

2.5. Autonomic

    2.5.1. Enuresis

    2.5.2. Periodic respiration, sleep apnea

    2.5.3. Painful erections

    2.5.4. . . .

    2.5.5. . . .

2.6. . . .

2.7. . . .

③ *3. Be able to classify and describe the sleep disorders associated with psychiatric conditions.*

③ *4. Be able to specify the relationship of medical disorders to the various stages of sleep.*

    Guide: Include:
    4.1. Myocardial infarction
    4.2. Duodenal ulcers
    4.3. . . .
    4.4. . . .

③ *5. Be able to state the relationship of various drugs to the stages of sleep.*

    Guide: Include:
    5.1. Their neurochemical mechanisms
    5.2. Effects of hypnotics, tranquilizers. and antidepressants on REM sleep
    5.3. Least "disrupting" sedatives
    5.4. Effects of long-term use of "sedating" medications
    5.5. . . .
    5.6 . . .

6. . . .

7. . . .

F. Experimental Psychopathology

i. Psychomimetic Agents

ENABLING OBJECTIVES

1. Be able to list three or four groups of euphorohallucinogenic compounds and to state for each:
④ *a. Chemical structure*
④ *b. Postulated mechanism of action*
③ *c. Complications*
③ *d. Description of psychological state, abnormalities of perception and behavior*
③ *e. Use (nontherapeutic and therapeutic)*
④ *f. Laboratory tests*

    Guide: Include:
    1.1. Indole alkaloids
    1.2. Piperidine derivatives
    1.3. Phenylethylamines
    1.4. Cannabinols
    1.5. . . .
    1.6. . . .

2. . . .

3. . . .

ii. Experimental Neurosis

ENABLING OBJECTIVES

③   *1. Be able to give evidence for the experimental production of neuroticlike states.*

　　Guide: Include:
　　1.1. Work on conflict and anxiety and the manifestations of these states in animals (e.g., Hebb, Pavlov, Gantt, Lidell, Masserman, Harlow)
　　1.2. Psychosomatic disorders (e.g., Mahl, Weiss, Porter)
　　1.3. Conflicts in humans (Luria)
　　1.4. Conditioning (Bykov)
　　1.5. Hypnotically induced emotions (Wittkower)
　　1.6. Starvation (Keys)
　　1.7. Stress (Funkenstein)
　　1.8. . . .
　　1.9. . . .
2. . . .
3. . . .

iii. Sensory Deprivation

ENABLING OBJECTIVES

③   *1. Be able to summarize the present state of scientific knowledge concerning sensory deprivation.*

　　Guide: Include:
　　1.1. Neurophysiological changes
　　1.2. Psychological and behavioral changes
　　1.3. Reversibility
　　1.4. Mechanism of action
　　1.5. Application to psychiatric practice and to other disciplines and vocations
　　1.6. . . .
　　1.7. . . .
2. . . .
3. . . .

iv. Sleep Deprivation

　　See Topic E, Sleep and Dreams.

G. Specialized Tests in Neurological Investigation

ENABLING OBJECTIVES

③   *1. For the commonly used "investigational" procedures in neuropsychiatry, be able to state:*

②	a. Indications and contraindications
②	b. Side effects
②	c. Complications (including probability of same)
②	d. Limitations
③	e. Methodology (briefly)
③	f. Indicators of pathology for major brain syndromes
③	g. Reliability and validity
③	h. Probability and meaning of false positives and false negatives

Guide: Include:
1.1. Electroencephalogram, including "special" techniques
1.2. Other techniques
    1.2.1. Air encephalograms
    1.2.2. Arteriograms
    1.2.3. Computer-assisted axial tomography
    1.2.4. CSF examination
    1.2.5. Echograms
    1.2.6. Radioisotope techniques (including computerized scanning)
    1.2.7. Skull X rays
    1.2.8. . . .
    1.2.9. . . .
1.3. . . .
1.4. . . .
2. . . .
3. . . .

H. Neurological Correlates of Specialized Procedures

ENABLING OBJECTIVES

1. For neuropsychiatric treatment procedures, be able to:

③	a. Describe methodology
③	b. List indications and contraindications
③	c. List and discuss possible complications
③	d. Discuss possible outcomes
④	e. Relate neurological (electophysiological) changes that occur during the procedures and state what is known about the mechanisms by which they work.

Guide: Include:
1.1. Biofeedback techniques
1.2. Hypnosis
1.3. . . .
1.4. . . .

2. Be able to state the neurological correlates of:

④	2.1. Auditory stimulation
④	2.2. Visual stimulation (e.g., evoked potentials)
④	2.3. Sensory deprivation

2.4. . . .
2.5. . . .
Include EEG changes and neurochemical changes where these are known.
3. . . .
4. . . .

Section IV.   Contributions of the Psychological Sciences
to Psychiatry

GENERAL PLAN

A. Motivation
B. Ethology
C. Cognition
   i. Intelligence
  ii. Language Development
D. Perception
E. General Systems Theory
F. Communications Theory

TERMINAL OBJECTIVE

To be capable of applying one's knowledge and understanding of psychological research concepts and findings to clinical assessment, diagnostic formulation, and therapeutic management.

A. Motivation

ENABLING OBJECTIVES

③   *1. Be able to cite evidence from animal and human experiments to sup-*
port or refute the importance of biological and learned factors to a com-
prehensive understanding of human motivation.

Guide: Include:
1.1. Largely biological mechanisms and concepts
    1.1.1. Homeostatic mechanisms (e.g., neuroendocrine, water and
       electrolyte)
    1.1.2. "Inborn" drives
       a. Hunger, cling, etc. (Bowlby)
       b. Hierarchy—hunger, security, affection, esteem, self-ac-
         tualization (Maslow)
       c. Concepts of instinct, appetitive behavior, curiosity, etc.
    1.1.3. Concepts of "activation" (e.g., imprinting, innate releasing
       mechanisms)
    1.1.4. "Conation." Neurophysiological basis for fear, anger, anx-
       iety, pleasure, arousal, other "drives"

        1.1.5. "State" of organism (e.g., deprivation, depression, intoxication)

        1.1.6. . . .

        1.1.7. . . .

    1.2. Largely "learned" mechanisms (psychological and social)

        1.2.1. Analytical (e.g., the unconscious, ego ideal, self-esteem)

        1.2.2. Learning theory (e.g., rewards and need reduction, conditioning, generalization, approach–avoidance, habit, cue)

        1.2.3. Other psychological factors—e.g., expectancy and value, aspiration, cognitive dissonance, perception, memory, novelty, boredom, difficulty, achievement, affiliation

        1.2.4. . . .

        1.2.5. . . .

   1.3. . . .

   1.4. . . .

③   2. *Be able to discuss critically the interrelationship of the factors mentioned in objective 1 as they pertain to clinical practice (where applicable).*

    Guide:

    2.1. On an individual level—with patients

    2.2. On a group level—with agencies and other human resource groups

③   3. *Be able to state briefly the significance to clinical psychiatric practice of some of the principal findings and hypotheses of more than five persons who have made major contributions to our present understanding of human motivation.*

    Guide: Among the workers that might be mentioned are:

    Adler, A.

    Allport, G.

    Bowlby, J.

    Dollard, J., and Miller, N.

    Festinger, L.

    Freud, S.

    Harlow, H.

    Lehrman, D. S.

    Maslow, A.

    Mowrer, O. H.

    Murray, H.

    Olds, J., and Milner, B.

   4. . . .

   5. . . .

B. Ethology

ENABLING OBJECTIVES

④   1. *Be able to state the major contributions of a minimum of five major contributors to the literature on ethology to our understanding of behavior.*

Guide: Among the workers that might be mentioned are:

Von Perneau (species-specific behavior)

Lorenz (innate releasing mechanism, imprinting, action-specific energy)

Tinbergen (displacement activity, hierarchy of appetitive behavior, and consumatory acts)

Hess (imprinting)

von Holst and others (on the neurophysiological basis of inborn behavior patterns)

Bowlby (infant behavior)

④   *2. Be able to define all the terms commonly used in this field.*

Guide: Include all terms in objective 1 above in addition to other current terms used in this field, such as: instinct, releasor, fixed action pattern, territoriality, agonistic behavior, sign stimuli, critical period.

③▽③△ *3. Be able to discuss briefly the possible significance of research in ethology to our understanding of human development, primary prevention, and clinical practice.*

③▽②△ *4. Be able to clearly define and differentiate psychology, ethology, and ecology.*

5. . . .

6. . . .

C. Cognition

Note: The following subtopics may be subsumed under the topic "cognition":

  i. Intelligence

 ii. Language Development

iii. Learning

 iv. Memory

  v. Motivation

 vi. Perception

All but i and ii are dealt with in other sections.

i. Intelligence (Thinking and Problem-Solving)

ENABLING OBJECTIVES

③▽③△ *1. Be able to state the basic tenets of current theoretical approaches toward a theory of "intelligence."*

Guide: Include:

1.1. The multifactorial approach (Americans such as Thorndike, Thurstone, Guilford), e.g., Guilford's three-dimensional structure of intellect model—operations, product, and content

1.2. Approaches centered around a postulated "g" or general factor (British scientists such as Spearman, Burt, Vernon), e.g., Philip

Vernon's hierarchical theory (with its group factors, verbal–numer-ical–educational and practical–mechanical– patial–physical)

1.3. The "structural" and "developmental" approach, e.g., Piaget (with an emphasis on assimilation, accommodation, equilibrium, staged development)

1.4. The combination approach (British—recently being developed), e.g., British Intelligence Scale (BIS) "Thurstone-like" factors + Guilford-like" processes or operations and contents + "Vernon-like" subscales + Piaget-like" developmental periods.

1.5. Overall approach: Hebbs's distinction between Intelligence A (ge-netic potentiality) and B (effective intelligence) and Vernon's Intelli-gence C (that which an intelligence test can test)

1.6. . . .

1.7. . . .

For each of the approaches listed above, be able to discuss briefly the following where they may apply:

a. Limitations of factor analysis

b. "Social usefulness" criterion in the incorporation of group factors

c. Effect of environmental factors on test performance (include culture)

d. Effect of motivation

e. . . .

f. . . .

2. *Be able to discuss, both with respect to general intelligence and with re-spect to specific factors in intelligence:*

③▽③△ 2.1. *The relationship of intelligence to achievement in theory and with respect to particular patients*

② 2.2. *The effect of acute and chronic brain syndromes on "intelligence"*

③ 2.3. *The relationship between intelligence and concept formation and "functional" mental disorders, e.g., schizophrenia, manic–depressive psychosis*

③ 2.4. *The effect of developmental "stage" on intelligence*

2.5. . . .

2.6. . . .

3. *For commonly used intelligence tests, be able to state (in addition to Section VIII.B):*

③ *a. Theoretical base*

③▽②△ *b. Limitations*

c. . . .

d. . . .

Guide: Include:

3.1. Stanford–Binet

3.2. WISC

3.3. WAIS

3.4. BIS (British Intelligence Scale)

3.5. Raven Progressive Matrices

3.6. . . .

3.7. . . .

④   *4. Using concepts of convergent and divergent (creative) thinking, be able to discuss critically the applicability (or lack thereof) of intelligence tests to measure potential for creative achievement.*

      5. . . .

      6. . . .

ii. Language Development

ENABLING OBJECTIVES

④   *1. Be able to discuss briefly the effects of "social" contact on language development.*

④   *2. Be able to state briefly the neurophysiological basis for verbal behavior.*

④   *3. Be able to list and discuss briefly the principles of language acquisition and its significance in the process of "thinking."*

      Guide: Include the work of:

      3.1. Whorf. B. L. (language basis for thinking)

      3.2. Bruner, J. S. (linguistics as basic for cognitive behavior)

      3.3. Skinner. B. F. (e.g., learning, imitation)

      3.4. Chomsky, N. (e.g., transformational grammar, deep structure)

      3.5. Piaget, J. [link concept formation (developmental) and language acquisition]

      3.6. . . .

      3.7. . . .

④   *4. Be able to state briefly the contributions of animal studies to our understanding of language acquisition.*

      Guide: Include:

      4.1. Gardner with chimp babies

      4.2. Marlor. P., with birds

      4.3. . . .

      4.4. . . .

      5. For the subject of disorders of speech and language, be able to:

④   *5.1. List the frequency of and describe each major type that may be found in a grade school population.*

③   *5.2.* List and describe (neurophysiological basis, clinical picture, probable outcome) the types of aphasia.*

②   *5.3.* State the key clinical differences among "organic" mutism, psychogenic mutism, and autism.*

②   *5.4.* Clinically distinguish schizophrenic language difficulties, aphasia, and dysphasia.*

            5.5. . . .

            5.6. . . .

      6. . . .

      7. . . .

---

*Although not reaching statistical significance at the .01 level, Canadians ranked each of these objectives one or two priority levels higher than Americans. Australians lay between the two.

D. Perception

ENABLING OBJECTIVES

④ *1. Be able to define perception and discuss current theoretical constructs.*

Guide: The following hypotheses and/or factors could be included in a theory of human perception:

1.1. Hypotheses centered around "first"-order mechanisms (objects as structures of elementary sensations), e.g., structuralist, analytic introspection (separation of raw sensation from memory), empiricist (learning theory)

1.2. Hypotheses centered around "second"-order variables (measured relationships between individual members), movement, ratios, gradients, and so on, and their relationship to unconscious interference

1.3. Hypotheses centered on "higher"-order variables—Gestalt (laws of organization of form, shape, space), causation

1.4. Hypotheses centered on the highest order of variables—social perception. (Inclusion here must not necessarily imply that the study of man's perceptual processes with respect to the "physical" world can provide "universal" laws that can be applied to psychosocial perception.) Socially produced distortions, socially altered recognition threshold (e.g., repression, preperceptual observation), non-verbal expression as cues to feeling and thinking, demand character of social perception, ambiguity of stimuli, strength of psychological set, needs and drives, and so on.

1.5. . . .

1.6. . . .

④ *2. Be able to discuss critically the effect of motivation (factors listed in topic A) on psychosocial perception.*

Guide:

2.1. Theoretically

2.2. With respect to a clinical case

③ *3. Be able to discuss succinctly the interrelationship of past experience, self esteem, and psychological defense mechanisms and perception.*

Guide:

3.1. Theoretically

3.2. With respect to a clinical case

④ *4. Be able to state briefly the present state of knowledge of the neurophysiological basis of perception.*

④ *5. Be able to state the relationship of a theory of perception to the methodology used in and the usefulness in clinical psychiatry of projective psychological tests.*

Guide: Include:

5.1. Rorschach

5.2. TAT

5.3. . . .

5.4. . . .

6. *Be able to comment briefly on the interrelationships of:*
   ④   6.1. *Field dependency to personality*
   ④   6.2. *Perception and attention to schizophrenia and manic–depressive disorder*
   ④ 7. *Be able to integrate your knowledge of perception into theories of personality development and psychopathology.*

8. . . .

9. . . .

E. General Systems Theory

ENABLING OBJECTIVES

③ 1. *"General systems theory attempts to create universal laws and hypotheses derived from, and equally applicable to, all branches of scientific endeavor." Be able to outline briefly what is meant by the term "general systems theory" and discuss the extent to which the foregoing statement is true insofar as its application to psychiatric theory and practice is concerned.*

④ 2. *Be able to define terms commonly used in systems theory.*

   Guide: Include:
   2.1.   Boundary
   2.2.   Cybernetics
   2.3.   Differentiation
   2.4.   Element
   2.5.   Feedback control
   2.6.   Gestalt
   2.7.   Input, output, and process
   2.8.   Interelement or intersector interaction
   2.9.   Intersystem generalization
   2.10. Level
   2.11. Mechanization
   2.12. Regression
   2.13. Stratification
   2.14. Structure
   2.15. System (open vs. closed)
   2.16. Time-dependent steady states
   2.17. Morphogenic
   2.18. . . .
   2.19. . . .

④ 3. *Be able to draw a schematic diagram of an open morphogenic system.*

4. *Noting, in particular, the terms listed in objective 2 above, be able to outline succinctly the contributions of general systems theory to:*

④   *4.1. Biological science (e.g., neuroendocrine system)*

④   *4.2. Understanding psychodynamics and the application of psycho-*
    therapy

④   *4.3. Understanding small groups and the application of group therapy,*
    family therapy, and "milieu" therapy

④   *4.4. Understanding large groups:*
        4.4.1. Community
        4.4.2. Culture

④   *4.5. The organization of human resources*
    4.6. . . .
    4.7. . . .
  5. . . .
  6. . . .

F. Communications Theory

ENABLING OBJECTIVES

④   *1. Be able to list the areas pertinent to psychiatric theory and practice and
subsumed under the rubric of communications theory.*

    Guide: This can include such far-reaching topics as:
    1.1.   Cybernetics
    1.2.   Information theory
    1.3.   Computers and other automatic devices
    1.4.   The genetic code
    1.5.   Neurochemistry
    1.6.   Neurophysiology
    1.7.   Language development
    1.8.   Ethology
    1.9.   Cognition
    1.10. Theories of interpersonal interactions (verbal and nonverbal)
    1.11. Extrasensory perception
    1.12. Propaganda
    1.13. The arts
    1.14. Decision-making systems
    1.15. Interviewing
    1.16. Psychotherapies
    1.17. . . .
    1.18. . . .

④   *2. See objectives in specific sections covering the topic areas referred to
above.*
  3. . . .
  4. . . .

Section V. Contributions of the Sociocultural Sciences to Psychiatry

GENERAL PLAN

A. Cultural Anthropology
   i. The Concept of Culture and Cultural Relativity
   ii. Cultural Variations in Marital Patterns and Family Structure
   iii. Cultural Change and Mental Health
B. Sociology, Ecology, and Social Psychiatry
   i. Concepts and Definitions
   ii. Social Class and Psychiatry
   iii. Important Ecological Factors Related to Psychiatric Disorders
   iv. The Sociology of Psychiatric Wards
C. Transcultural Psychiatry
   i. Variations in the Forms of Psychiatric Disorders According to Culture
   ii. Variations in the Epidemiology of Psychiatric Disorders According to Culture

A. Cultural Anthropology

i. The Concept of Culture and Cultural Relativity

TERMINAL OBJECTIVE

To attain an understanding of some of the various concepts of culture and of the idea that cultures have arrived at a variety of greatly diverse solutions to the problems of survival and the achievement of satisfaction.

ENABLING OBJECTIVES

③   *1. Be able to list and discuss some of the universal biological, psychological, and social needs of human beings and to compare and contrast the means by which your own cultural groups meets these needs with the means by which one or two other cultural groups do so.*
③   *2. Be able to discuss the concept of cultural relativity:*

   Guide:
   2.1. Referring to such specific phenomena as hallucinations, paranoidal thinking, and dissociational (trance) states
   2.2. Differentiating between egodystonic (conflicts) and egosyntonic behavior and delineating in particular the two broad categories of egosyntonic behavior: socially deviant and culturally ritualized
   2.3. Comparing attitudes of contrasting cultures to such behaviors as transvestitism, nudity, premarital sexual behavior, and cannabis use

2.4. . . .
2.5. . . .
3. . . .
4. . . .

ii. Cultural Variations in Marital Patterns and Family Structure

TERMINAL OBJECTIVE

To learn the range and diversity of marital and family patterns across cultures and the ecological forces that may determine them.

ENABLING OBJECTIVES

④ 1. *Polygyny, polyandry, and monogamy are the major marital patterns to be found in world cultures. Be able to list the following major characteristics for each:*
   1.1. *Structure*
   1.2. *Relative frequency*
   1.3. *Possible ecological determinants*
   1.4. *Advantages and disadvantages*
   1.5. *Specific culture(s) in which practiced*
   1.6. . . .
   1.7. . . .
③ 2. *Be able to discuss the effect of social contexts on attitude and behavior, with particular attention to:*
   2.1. *"Deviation from the culturally dominant role," particularly with respect to the changing role of women in North America*
   2.2. *Violence and antisocial behavior*
   2.3. . . .
   2.4. . . .
④ 3. *Be able to list the major distinguishing characteristics of the following family forms: matrilineal, patrilocal extended, Western nuclear.*
③ 4. *Be able to compare and contrast the attitudes of immigrant groups (e.g., Italian, Greek, Ukrainian) with those of the Anglo-Saxon majority with regard to:*
   4.1. *Dating practices of adolescent daughters*
   4.2. *Authority of father*
   4.3. *Role of mother*
   4.4. *Importance of education for children*
   4.5. . . .
   4.6. . . .
5. . . .
6. . . .

iii. Cultural Change and Mental Health

TERMINAL OBJECTIVE

To have an awareness of some of the research concepts related to the mental health aspects of cultural change and migration.

ENABLING OBJECTIVES

③▽③△ *1. Be able to describe studies linking cultural change or migration to changes in mental health.*
③▽②△ *2. Be able to list major changes of psychiatric relevance taking place in our own culture today.*
    3. For each of the changes listed above, discuss:
③   *3.1. Mental health implications*
③   *3.2. Segments of the population most likely to be affected*
③   *3.3. Whether changes are likely (in your view) to result in poorer mental health*
③   *3.4. Methods for prevention where appropriate*
       3.5. . . .
       3.6. . . .
    4. . . .
    5. . . .

B. Sociology, Ecology, and Social Psychiatry

i. Concepts and Definitions

TERMINAL OBJECTIVE

To become familiar with some of the main concepts and terms used by sociology when considering psychiatric phenomena.

ENABLING OBJECTIVES

③   *1. Be able to define the following terms and discuss the relevance of each for psychiatry:*
       1.1. Status and role
       1.2. Deviant behavior
       1.3. Sick role
       1.4. Social disintegration
       1.5. Census tract
       1.6. Institution
       1.7. Protestant ethic
       1.8. Anomie
       1.9. Alienation

    1.10. . . .
    1.11. . . .

③   2. *Be able to give three examples of common "role conflicts" that might have psychiatric implications.*

③   3. *Be able to discuss the relationship of the following commonly recorded epidemiological factors to frequency or type, or both, of psychiatric disorder:*
    3.1. Age
    3.2. Sex
    3.3. Marital status
    3.4. Religion
    3.5. . . .
    3.6. . . .
  4. . . .
  5. . . .

ii. Social Class and Psychiatry

TERMINAL OBJECTIVE

To attain an understanding of what is meant by social class and how social class position may be related to psychiatric disorders, psychiatric treatment, and the attitudes of the psychiatrist.

ENABLING OBJECTIVES

③   1. *Be able to define social class and list the information required to assign an individual to a class position.*

③   2. *Hollingshead's social class categories have been widely used in social psychiatric studies. Be able to describe the distinguishing features of each of the categories.*

②   3. *Be able to state how social class is related to the frequency, diagnosis, and treatment of psychiatric disorders.*

③   4. *Be able to discuss the methods by which a psychiatric clinic can adapt its operation to give adequate service to patients of different social classes.*
  5. . . .
  6. . . .

iii. Important Ecological Factors Related to Psychiatric Disorders

TERMINAL OBJECTIVE

To become familiar with research findings concerning relationships between various ecological factors and differential rates (and patterns) of psychiatric disorders.

ENABLING OBJECTIVES

③   1. *In a variety of urban studies, area of residence has been found to be related to frequency and type of psychiatric disorders. Be able to discuss the possible reasons for these findings.*

    Guide:
    1.1. Be able to discuss the environmental factors, both physical and social, that influence the incidence and prevalence of major psychiatric syndromes, e.g., the origin vs. downward drift polemic with schizophrenia.
    1.2. Be able to discuss factors in the physical environment that affect the incidence and prevalence of antisocial behavior.
    1.3. . . .
    1.4. . . .

③   2. *Be able to discuss the importance to psychiatric theory and practice of major epidemiological studies.*

    Guide: For subobjectives 1.1 and 1.2 above, be able to list the goals and major findings of the following studies:
    a. Faris and Dunham: Mental Disorders in Urban Areas
    b. Hollingshead and Redlich: Social Class and Mental Illness
    c. Cummings and Cummings: Closed Ranks
    d. Srole *et al.*: Midtown Manhattan Study
    e. Kornhauser: Mental Health of the Industrial Worker
    f. Leighton: Stirling County Study
    g. Odegaard: Emigration and Insanity (a study of Norwegians in Minnesota
    h. . . .
    i. . . .

    3. . . .
    4. . . .

iv. The Sociology of Psychiatric Wards

TERMINAL OBJECTIVE

    To attain an awareness of some of the studies and findings concerning the social systems of psychiatric wards and their implications for reform.

ENABLING OBJECTIVES

③   1. *Be able to list and discuss some of the findings of sociologists (and others) who have admitted themselves anonymously to psychiatric wards.*

③   2. *Be able to state the features of "hospital neurosis" (nestling syndrome, hospitalitis, institutional neurosis) and discuss its genesis.*

③   3. *Be able to state and discuss the contributions of social psychiatric studies such as those of Caudill and Goffman to our understanding of mental hospitals.*

4. . . .

5. . . .

C. Transcultural Psychiatry

i. Variations in the Forms of Psychiatric Disorders According to Culture

TERMINAL OBJECTIVE

To have an awareness that all cultures generate psychiatric disorders, but that their forms may vary from culture to culture in a way that is linked to cultural symbols, belief systems, or modal personalities.

ENABLING OBJECTIVES

1. Be able to:

③   *1.1. Define a culture-bound syndrome.*

④   *1.2. Describe four syndromes that have been regarded as examples of it.*

③   *1.3. Discuss the adequacy of the concept itself.*

④   *1.4. Discuss whether such syndromes fit our diagnostic classification systems or not.*

    1.5. . . .

    1.6. . . .

2. . . .

3. . . .

ii. Variations in the Epidemiology of Psychiatric Disorders According to Culture*

TERMINAL OBJECTIVE

To learn that the prevalence, age of onset, duration, and outcome of psychiatric disorders may vary across cultures and that variations are often best explained in cultural terms.

ENABLING OBJECTIVES

③▽③▲ *1. Be able to list variations in prevalence, ages of onset, duration, and outcome of psychiatric disorders among different cultures.*

    1.1. Be able to discuss possible cultural explanations for these differences. Include:

    1.1.1. Suicide

    1.1.2. Schizophrenia

*See also Section XX.C.

> 1.1.3. *Depression*
> 1.1.4. *. . .*
> 1.1.5. *. . .*
> 2. *. . .*
> 3. *. . .*

Section VI. Child and Adolescent Psychiatry

GENERAL PLAN

A. Child Psychiatry
   i. Child Development
   ii. Syndromes in Child Psychiatry
   iii. Treatment in Child Psychiatry
   iv. Adolescence and Its Problems
   v. Psychiatric Problems of the Child and Family
B. Mental Retardation
C. Genetics

A. Child Psychiatry*

i. Child Development

TERMINAL OBJECTIVE

To become familiar with some of the major theories of child development.

ENABLING OBJECTIVES

1. *Be able to list the major contributions that each of the following workers has made toward a theory of child development:*
    | | 1.1. | *Birch* | *(nutrition)* |
    |②| 1.2 | *Bowlby, J.* | *(maternal deprivation)* |
    |③▽②△| 1.3 | *Chess, S.* | *(temperament)* |
    | | 1.4. | *Eisenberg, L.* | *(social system roles)* |
    |②| 1.5. | *Erikson, E.* | *(stages of development)* |
    |④| 1.6. | *Fraiberg, S. H.* | *(stages of development)* |
    |②| 1.7. | *Freud, S.* | *(stages of development)* |
    |②| 1.8. | *Freud, A.* | *(mechanisms of defense)* |
    |③| 1.9. | *Gesell* | *(stages of development)* |
    |③| 1.10. | *Harlow, H.* | *(experimental)* |
    |②| 1.11. | *Piaget, J.* | *(cognition)* |
    | | 1.12. | *Rutter, M.* | *(separation, hyperactivity)* |

*Although not reaching a .01 level of significance, there was a definite trend for Canadians and Australians to give a slightly higher priority ranking to objectives in this section.

③   *1.13. Skinner, B. F.   (learning theory)*
③   *1.14. Spitz, R. A.   (hospitalism)*
③   *1.15. Winnicott   (transitional objects)*
        1.16. . . .
        1.17. . . .
   2. For each of the theoretical approaches to understanding the child listed below:
      a. Be able to state and describe the tenets on which the theory is based.
      b. Using objective 1 above as a guide, list the major contributions to each theoretical approach.
③   *2.1. Psychoanalytic theory*
③   *2.2. Cognitive theory*
③   *2.3. Learning theory*
③   *2.4. Attachment theory and general systems theory*
③   *2.5. Constitutional theory*
        2.6. . . .
        2.7. . . .
③ *3. Be able to derive and list the essential (major) concepts held in common by members of each of the major developmental theoretical groups.*
② *4. Be able to make up a chart that relates the milestones of physical, emotional, and social development to the age ranges within which these milestones are most likely to occur, including in the chart, as a minimum:*
      4.1. Developmental tasks (Erickson)
      4.2. Stages of psychosexual development (Freud)
      4.3. Stages of cognitive development (Piaget)
      4.4. Stages of speech development
      4.5. Fine and gross motor development
      4.6. The developmental problems that are likely to occur at each stage
      4.7. . . .
      4.8. . . .
   5. . . .
   6. . . .

ii. Syndromes in Child Psychiatry

TERMINAL OBJECTIVE

   To become familiar with the major psychiatric syndromes encountered in children and adolescents.

ENABLING OBJECTIVES

②* *1. Be able to list the syndromes about which a psychiatrist should have a working knowledge. Use DSM, ICD, or GAP report.*

*All ratings marked by asterisk were ▽ □ △ , but not to a level of .005 significance.

2. *Be able to describe each of the syndromes listed in objective 1 above under the following headings:*

②*   2.1.   *Definition*
②*   2.2.   *Description*
②   2.3.   *Classification*
②   2.4.   *Etiology (including psychopathogenesis)*
②   2.5.   *Psychopathology (including pathophysiology where appropriate)*
②*   2.6.   *Clinical course*
②*   2.7.   *Clinical management*
②   2.8.   *Prognosis*
       2.9.   . . .
       2.10. . . .

③   3. *Be able to discuss the contributions of four major authors to an understanding of psychosis in childhood.*

Guide: Authors that might be included are:
3.1. Kanner, L.
3.2. Mahler, M.
3.3. Rutter, M.
3.4. Creak (British Working Party)
3.5. . . .
3.6. . . .

4. . . .
5. . . .

iii. Treatment in Child Psychiatry

TERMINAL OBJECTIVES

1. To become familiar with the major forms of therapeutic intervention available within child psychiatry.
2. To develop some rationale for the selective use of each of these forms of therapy.

ENABLING OBJECTIVES

②   1. *Be able to list the following therapeutic techniques commonly used in the treatment of children and their families:*
       1.1. *Crisis intervention (see Section IX for details)*
       1.2. *Counseling of parents, child, or both*
       1.3. *Environmental manipulation*
       1.4. *Chemotherapy (see Section XIV for details)*
       1.5. *Forms of psychotherapeutic intervention (see Section XVI for details)*
             1.5.1. *Planned brief psychotherapy*

---

*All ratings marked by asterisk were Ⅴ①Δ, but not to a level of .005 significance.

       1.5.2. Individual psychotherapy with child or adolescent

       1.5.3. Individual psychotherapy with child or adolescent combined with casework (or counseling or psychotherapy) with parents or family

       1.5.4. Family therapy

       1.5.5. Group therapy

       1.5.6. . . .

       1.5.7. . . .

    1.6. Behavior therapy (see Section XV for details)

    1.7. Milieu therapy

    1.8. . . .

    1.9. . . .

2. *Be able to discuss each of the treatment approaches listed in objective 1 above under the following headings:*

  ②   *2.1. Definition*

  ②   *2.2. Description*

  ③   *2.3. Classification*

  ②   *2.4. Indications*

  ②   *2.5. Contraindications*

  ②   *2.6. Side (and toxic) effects*

  ②   *2.7. Efficacy*

  ③   *2.8. Theoretical method of action*

       2.9. . . .

       2.10. . . .

3. *. . .*

4. *. . .*

iv. Adolescence and Its Problems

TERMINAL OBJECTIVE

To achieve an understanding of adolescence as a developmental stage, and to apply this understanding to an understanding of the psychopathology of adolescence.

ENABLING OBJECTIVES

①   1. *Be able to define adolescence.*

    Guide: What are the major parameters in which change is occurring?

①   2. *Be able to list and describe the major developmental tasks of adolescence.*

①   3. *Be able to list and discuss problems commonly experienced by adolescents related to failure to successfully achieve each of the major developmental tasks listed in objective 2 above.*

①   4. *Be able to discuss the difficulties that parents of adolescents frequently have in relation to their teenagers' achievement of each of these major developmental tasks.*

①   *5. Be able to discuss the clinical management of the psychiatric problems
     of the adolescent and his family.*

> *Guide:* Include:
> 5.1. A discussion of the indications and contraindications of particular
>   forms of treatment
> 5.2. Some discussion of differences in the treatment process arising be-
>   cause of the patient's being an adolescent
> 5.3. . . .
> 5.4. . . .

     6. . . .
     7. . . .

v. Psychiatric Problems of the Child and Family*

TERMINAL OBJECTIVE

To understand disturbance in a child as it affects and is affected by the
equilibrium of the family system.

ENABLING OBJECTIVES

③   *1. Be able to describe both major classic and current contributions to our
     knowledge of the "family" and family therapy.*

> *Guide:* Include the work of:
> 1.1. Ackerman, N.
> 1.2. Jackson, D.
> 1.3. Haley, J., and Satir, V.
> 1.4. Lidz, T.
> 1.5. Bowen, M.
> 1.6. Wynne, L.
> 1.7. Epstein, N.
> 1.8. . . .
> 1.9. . . .

     *2. Be able to describe the role that each of the following concepts or the-
     ories has in family therapy theory:*
③   *2.1.   The concept of family homeostatis (effects of stress on)*
③   *2.2.   Psychoanalytic theory*
③   *2.3.   Role therapy*
③   *2.4.   Systems theory*
③   *2.5.   Communications theory*
③   *2.6.   The concept of schism and skew*
③   *2.7.   The concept of pseudomutuality*
③   *2.8.   The concept of double bind*
     2.9.   . . .
     2.10. . . .

*See also Section XVI.

3. . . .
4. . . .

B. Mental Retardation

TERMINAL OBJECTIVE

To become aware that the problem of mental retardation involves the interplay of biological, psychological, social, and cultural factors, and that prevention and treatment must take account of this interplay.

ENABLING OBJECTIVES*

1. Become skilled in the differential diagnosis of:
②   *1.1. Mental retardation from other psychopathological syndromes*
②   *1.2. Mental retardation from "normative" development*
④ *2. Be able to interpret and communicate with nonverbal children.*
③ *3. Be able to assess and counter negative feelings in relation to mentally retarded patients and families.*
④ *4. Be able to demonstrate an ability to fulfill the combined role of an interdisciplinary coordinator consultant and direct therapist.*

> *Guide:* Participate actively in the following learning situations:
> 4.1. A diagnostic clinic for the mentally retarded
> 4.2. Observation of retarded children in natural surroundings
> 4.3. Joint interviewing with supervisors in clinic and "community"
> 4.4. Exposure to the spectrum of mental retardation syndromes
> 4.5. Family and staff conferences
> 4.6. Utilization of all community resources in an ongoing fashion with a patient for whom you are responsible
> 4.7. Parent education programs with respect to all aspects of prevention: primary. secondary. and tertiary
> 4.8. . . .
> 4.9. . . .

③ *5. Be able to discuss the etiological determinants of mental retardation.*

> *Guide:*
> 5.1. Discuss the biological, psychological. social. and cultural factors that may be involved and the interactions among them.
> 5.2. Show a working knowledge of the epidemiology of mental retardation.
> 5.3. . . .
> 5.4. . . .

6. . . .
7. . . .

*Although not reaching a .005 level of significance, for all objectives in this section the Canadian ranking is one level higher than the American. The Australian falls between the two.

C. Genetics

TERMINAL OBJECTIVE

To learn about the basic principles of genetics necessary for the understanding of the hereditary basis of cognitive and affective disorders, and to be able to participate in genetic counseling with regard to such disorders.

ENABLING OBJECTIVES

③▽③△* *1. Be able to briefly discuss cytogenetics.*

Guide: Describe:
1.1. Sex chromatin
1.2. Chromosome techniques
1.3. Turner's syndrome XO
1.4. Klinefelter's XXY
1.5. XYY
1.6. Down's syndrome
1.7. . . .
1.8. . . .

③ *2. Be able to briefly discuss biochemical genetics.*

Guide: Describe:
2.1. Mutation
2.2. DNA
2.3. Inborn errors including PKU, porphyria
2.4. . . .
2.5. . . .

③ *3. Be able to describe genotypes and phenotypes and give one example of each of the following simple patterns of inheritance:*
3.1. Sex-linked recessive
3.2. Autosomal "intermediate"

③ *4. Be able to discuss the use of the "twin method" in attempting to resolve the heredity vs. environment polemic.*

③ *5. Be able to discuss briefly the genetic basis of mental retardation, with particular attention to:*
5.1. Mental deficiency due to a dominant gene
5.2. Mental deficiency due to a single recessive gene
5.3. Mental deficiency associated with chromosomal abnormalities
5.4. Mental deficiency due to an undetermined genetic mechanism
5.5. . . .
5.6. . . .

② *6. Be able to discuss briefly the genetic basis of psychiatric syndromes.*

Guide: Include. where applicable:
6.1. The schizophrenic disorders
6.2. The affective disorders

*Level of significance .008.

6.3. The neuroses, including anxiety and somatoform and dissociative disorders

6.4. Personality disorders

6.5. The psychosexual disorders

6.6. Sleep disorders

6.7. ...

6.8. ...

③ 7. *Be able to draft family geneologies using conventional symbols for sex, affected member, carrier, twin, proband generation, and so on.*

④ 8. *Having had experience in actively participating as a psychiatric consultant to a genetic counselor, be able to provide risk figures to families for common psychiatric and mental retardation syndromes.*

④ 9. *Be able to state existing mandatory and permissive legislation regarding genetic counseling.*

10. ...

11. ...

Section VII.   Theories of Personality and Psychopathology

GENERAL PLAN*

A. Personality Development and the Life Cycle
Relevance: Age norms, regression in illness, psychogenetic diagnosis

B. Personality Organization and Component Functions
Relevance: Cross-sectional clinical assessment, psychodynamic diagnosis

C. Homeostasis, Motivation, Conflict, and Symptomatology
Relevance: Psychodynamic diagnosis, treatment planning

D. Phenomenology, Nosology, and General Psychopathology
Relevance: Clinical assessment and differential diagnosis, treatment planning, prognosis, epidemiology

TERMINAL OBJECTIVE

To be able to present an integrated theory of personality and its development and to integrate the biological, psychological, and social components.

A. Personality Development and the Life Cycle

ENABLING OBJECTIVES

③ 1. *Be able to outline practical age norms for physical and neuromuscular capabilities, cognitive and conceptual capacities, expected drives and*

*These areas are not necessarily mutually exclusive, and the placing of an objective in one section as opposed to another becomes, at times, arbitrary. See also, for example, Sections II, Normality and Normal Psychosexual Development; VI, Child and Adolescent Psychiatry; and XIX, Gender and Psychiatry.

motivational conflicts, and their resolution at various stages of life (see Section VI.A.i, objective 4).

② 2. *Be able to outline the nature of the family of origin and the family of procreation and their part in the patient's life, together with the patient's changing roles and relationships in relation to these families.*

Guide: Include:

2.1. See Section VI.A.v, objective 2.

2.2. A brief account of the significance of mother and parents based on the need for interpersonal relationships (bonding, *not* sexuality)

2.3. An account of the process of internalization of the parents by learning and the formation of internal structure, including:

2.3.1. Superego, ego, id

2.3.2. Self

2.3.3. Parent, adult and child

2.4. . . .

2.5. . . .

③ 3. *Be able to state the contributions of major authors to our conceptual understanding of human development.*

Guide: Include:

3.1.   Abraham, K.

3.2.   Benedict, R.

3.3.   Chess, S.

3.4.   Erikson, E.

3.5.   Freud, A.

3.6.   Freud, S.

3.7.   Gesell, A.

3.8.   Jaspers, K.

3.9.   Piaget, J.

3.10. Spock, B.

3.11. Sullivan, H. S.

3.12. . . .

3.13. . . .

② 4. *Be able to present a comprehensive case history for each of the following: neurosis, functional psychosis, organic brain syndrome, personality disorder, psychophysiological disorder, and a transient situational disturbance.*

Guide: For each, identify and conceptualize:

4.1.   Family constellation and prenatal history

4.2.   Developmental sequence of major changes in the patient through infancy, childhood, puberty, adolescence, young adulthood, middle life, and old age (as far as applicable)

4.3.   Significant conflicts at each stage, with their resolution or lack of resolution, and significant developmental traumata and arrests

4.4.   The level of developmental or psychosexual function achieved by the patient prior to breakdown

4.5. Regression to earlier modes of functioning

4.6. The repetitive "characterological" behavioral (coping) patterns including "transactional" patterns of relating that the patient exhibits under stress

4.7. The historical, transactional, and psychodynamic origins of such behavior patterns

4.8. The significance of the early "concepts of self" and "ideal self" and relate them to psychological growth and development

4.9. . . .

4.10. . . .

5. . . .

6. . . .

B. Personality Organization and Component Functions

ENABLING OBJECTIVES

② 1. *Be able to state and give an account of the basic concepts of the psychoanalytic theory of personality structure and development.*

Guide: This account should include knowledge of:

1.1. Psychic structure, i.e., id, ego, superego

1.2. The pattern of psychological development from infancy to maturity

1.3. Psychological defense mechanisms

1.4. The basic concepts of "ego psychology"

1.5. The theory of symptom formation giving rise to neurotic and character disorders

1.6. How the conflict between internal structures as a result of frustration of interpersonal needs in childhood may lead to conflict solutions based on learning from the parents by identification (defenses)

1.7. The significance of self esteem for conflict solution and interpersonal relations

1.8. The postulated mechanism for psychotic symptom formation

1.9. The basic contributions of:

1.9.1. Bowlby, J.

1.9.2. Erikson, E.

1.9.3. Freud, A.

1.9.4. Freud, S.

1.9.5. Hartman, H., *et al.*

1.9.6. Klein, M.

1.9.7. . . .

1.9.8. . . .

1.10. . . .

1.11. . . .

④   *2. Be able to state the basic concepts of existential theories of personality structure and development.*

       Guide: Relate some of the basic contributions of such persons as Binswanger, Jaspers, and Rollo May.

③   *3. Be able to state briefly the contributions of major authors to a theory of personality structure.*

       Guide: Include:
       3.1. Adler, A.
       3.2. Berne, E.
       3.3. Fromm, E.
       3.4. Horney, K.
       3.5. Masserman, J.
       3.6. Meyer, A.
       3.7. Sullivan, H. S.
       3.8. . . .
       3.9. . . .

③   *4. Be able to state, using clinical examples, the significance of the "concept of self" in perception and motivation and relate this "structural entity" to ego states.*

③   *5. Be able to define and explain the terms commonly used in describing personality structures and processes.*

       Guide:
       5.1.   Drive
       5.2.   Avoidance
       5.3.   Value system
       5.4.   Id
       5.5.   Ego
       5.6.   Superego
       5.7.   Basic and acquired need
       5.8.   Operant and classical conditioning
       5.9.   Reinforcement
       5.10. Organ conditioning
       5.11. Learning
       5.12. Communication
       5.13. Cognition
       5.14. Memory
       5.15. Memory trace
       5.16. Ego states (parent, adult, child)
       5.17. Script
       5.18. Gestalt
       5.19. Basic existential position
       5.20. Defense mechanism
       5.21. . . .
       5.22. . . .

③   6. *Be able to state the major contributions of cognitive and learning theorists.*

      Guide:
      6.1. Catell, R. B.
      6.2. Eysenck, H. J.
      6.3. Lazarus, A. A.
      6.4. Pavlov, I.
      6.5. Piaget, P.
      6.6. Skinner, B. F.
      6.7. . . .
      6.8. . . .

③   7. *Be able to discuss the factors underlying aggressive behavior.*

      Guide:
      7.1. Biological factors
      7.2. Result of frustration in childhood
      7.3. Secondary phenomena of aggression, guilt, depression, and self destruction
      7.4. . . .
      7.5. . . .

    8. *Be able to discuss:*

③   8.1. *Sexuality as a primary need* separate *from the need for bonding*
②   8.2. *Pathological sexual attitudes as an outcome of interpersonal conflicts*
③   8.3. *The use of sex for ulterior motives:*
        8.3.1. *Support of self-esteem*
        8.3.2. *Revenge for interpersonal frustrations*
        8.3.3. *Sexual biases as reflected in current theories of personality structure and function*
        8.3.4. . . .
        8.3.5. . . .
      8.4. . . .
      8.5. . . .
    9. . . .
   10. . . .

C. Homeostasis, Motivation, Conflict, and Symptomatology

ENABLING OBJECTIVES

    1. *Be able to:*

②   1.1. *Psychodynamically differentiate a conversion reaction from a psychophysiological disorder.*
②   1.2. *Relate how adjustment or maladjustment of a brain-damaged patient may be dependent on coping mechanisms and how these mech-*

*anisms can either minimize or increase the patient's confusional
deficit.*

④   *1.3. Use dreams to monitor progress of a toxic state or the physician-
patient relationship, or both.*

    1.4. . . .

    1.5. . . .

①   2. *Be able to outline the mental mechanisms commonly and crucially involved in both psychotic and nonpsychotic mental disorders, including:*

   Guide:

   2.1. Depression and suicide

   2.2. Conversion and amnestic reactions

   2.3. Paranoid conditions

   2.4. Obsessive–compulsive personality and neurosis

   2.5 Anxiety states

   2.6. Hallucinosis and dreaming

      2.6.1. Include "defense" mechanisms such as repression, projec-
tion, and reaction formation.

      2.6.2. . . .

      2.6.3. . . .

   2.7. . . .

   2.8. . . .

③   3. *Be able to demonstrate the ability to use learning theory in understanding the formation and maintenance of symptoms, and in planning effective treatment strategies.*

②   4. *Since personality theory relates crucially to clinical psychiatry in the area
of motivation and adaptation, be able to demonstrate detailed knowledge and practical application of concepts of stress, anxiety, adaptation,
motivational conflict, the breakdown of adaptation, the mental mechanisms involved, and the pathways of symptom formation.*

③   5. *Be able to show how a patient uses repetitive characterological transactional patterns of relating to maintain a known equilibrium (existential
position).*

④   6. *Be able to state the manner in which, and the mechanisms by which, a
patient prevents himself from experiencing (awareness of) the "gestalt"
(self-in-the-world or self context) and from adequately separating "figure and ground."*

①   7. *Be able to demonstrate an integrated knowledge of personality structures, processes, and functions by doing case formulations that show
clearly the biological, psychological, and social components of the contributing, precipitating, and sustaining factors for the "behavioral" (including thought and emotion) patterns observed and related.*

   Guide: In doing so:

   7.1. Refer to major theoretical constructs, e.g., analytical, existential,
behaviorist.

7.2. Integrate endogenous and exogenous factors:
    7.2.1. Endogenous factors
        a. Inborn
           Innate needs
           Biological and acquired drives
           Inborn temperament
           Innate releasing mechanisms
           Cognitive ability
           . . .

           . . .

        b. Learned
           Conditioned responses
           Values (conscience, superego)
           Family images (parent, ego ideal)
           "Games and rackets"
           Coping repertoire (social skills, ego defenses)
           . . .

           . . .

        c. Mixed
           Problem-solving ability
           Emotional lability
           Communicational abilities
           "Primary gains"
           . . .

           . . .

    7.2.2. Exogenous factors
           External pressures (e.g., social realities, constraints, frustrations, object loss)
           External resources (e.g., significant others)
           Reinforcing factors [e.g., morbid (secondary) gains]
7.3. Summarize external and internal changes causing a shift in the homeostatic psychic balance.
7.4. Note the key mechanisms being employed to maintain homeostasis and how they relate to the patient's syndromes.
7.5. Note the importance of "self concept," "existential position," and "life script" in maintaining the characterological patterns of the patient's behavior.
7.6. . . .
7.7. . . .
8. . . .
9. . . .

D. Phenomenology, Nosology, and General Psychopathology

ENABLING OBJECTIVES

1. *Be able to give a succinct and accurate account of, and relate to clinical problems:*

②   *1.1. The present official psychiatric nomenclature, DSM or ICD, and the reasons for their major and detailed divisions*

③   *1.2. Basic psychiatric phenomenology*

        Guide: Identify contributions of:
        1.2.1.   Beck, A.
        1.2.2.   Bleuler, E.
        1.2.3.   Grinker, R.
        1.2.4.   Hecker, E.
        1.2.5.   Jaspers, K.
        1.2.6.   Kahlbaum, K.
        1.2.7.   Kraepelin, E.
        1.2.8.   Schneider, K.
        1.2.9.   Shapiro, D.
        1.2.10. . . .
        1.2.11. . . .

④   *1.3. An existential approach to the patient's experience*

        Guide: Identify contributions by:
        1.3.1.   Binswanger, L.
        1.3.2.   Fromm-Reichmann, F.
        1.3.3.   Frankl, V.
        1.3.4.   Laing, R. D.
        1.3.5.   Marcuse, H.
        1.3.6.   Sartre, J.
        1.3.7.   Rogers, C.
        1.3.8.   Sullivan, H.
        1.3.9.   . . .
        1.3.10. . . .

①   *2. Be able to define, accurately and operationally, commonly used terms such as:*

        2.1. Agnosia*
        2.2. Ambivalence
        2.3. Aphasia
        2.4. Autism
        2.5. Blocking
        2.6. Catastrophic reaction
        2.7. Circumstantiality
        2.8. Clang associations
        2.9. Compulsion
        2.10. Conation
        2.11. Confabulation
        2.12. Déjà vu, fausse reconnaissance
        2.13. Delirium
        2.14. Delusion

---

*Agnosia (nominal, syntactical, semantic, jargon, paraphasia).

Section VIII.   Psychiatric Assessment

GENERAL PLAN

A. The Interview
B. Assessment in Psychiatry
C. Nosology

A. The Interview

TERMINAL OBJECTIVE

To attain competence in interview methods:
1. The Diagnostic Interview—to assess personality, behavior, and the mental state.
2. The Therapeutic Interview—to assist a person to set "contracts," change behavior, feeling, thinking, and understanding.
3. The Epidemiological Interview—to obtain from the subject objective

facts that, as informant, he knows about, but the interviewer does not, e.g., social surveys.

4. . . .

ENABLING OBJECTIVES

①   *1. Be able to list the headings subsumed under the psychiatric assessment and to discuss in detail the type and the use of information gathered in each of these areas for each of the categories in a classification of mental disorders (ICD or DSM).*
Indirect Examination

Guide:
1.1. Identification profile. referral source. and recent involvements with other agencies
1.2. Chief complaints or problem list
1.3. History of present illness
1.4. Past medical (includes psychiatric) history
1.5. Functional inquiry
1.6. Family history (of origin)
1.7. Educational history
1.8. Occupational history
1.9. Socialization history
1.10. Marital and common-law history
1.11. Sexual history
1.12. Leisure time activities
1.13. Living arrangements and financial situation
1.14. "Legal" history
1.15. Assets and resources
1.16. Premorbid personality
1.17. . . .
1.18. . . .
Direct Examination

Guide:
①   1.19. Physical (includes neurological) examination
1.20. Mental status examination
1.21. Other investigations:
      1.21.1. Biological
      1.21.2. Psychological
      1.21.3. Educational
      1.21.4. Vocational
      1.21.5. . . .
      1.21.6. . . .
1.22. . . .
1.23. . . .

②   2. *Define the structure of an interview.*

       Guide:
       2.1. Beginning
       2.2. Body
       2.3. Termination

②   3. *List the qualities of an interviewer.*

       Guide:
       3.1. Empathy
       3.2. Rapport
       3.3. Congruence
       3.4. . . .
       3.5. . . .

③   4. *List current theoretical approaches to interviewing.*

       Guide:
       4.1. Psychological, e.g., Freud, S., Sullivan, H.
       4.2. Behavioral, e.g., Wolpe, J.
       4.3. Family
       4.4. . . .
       4.5. . . .

①   5. *List the difficulties an interviewer might encounter.*

       Guide:
       5.1. In the patient (e.g., resistance)
       5.2. In himself or herself (e.g., countertransference)
       5.3. . . .
       5.4. . . .

③   6. *Be able to state contributions to interviewing techniques by the representatives of various schools of thought.*

②   7. *Be able to:*
       7.1. Define the meaning of empathy, intuition, and sensitivity.
       7.2. Demonstrate these attributes in the interview situation.

①   8. *Be able to demonstrate in the interview situation that your awareness of your own feelings and "attitudes" has positively influenced your own ability to:*
       8.1. Gain rapport.
       8.2. Correctly identify significant problem areas.
       8.3. Initiate treatment.
       8.4. . . .
       8.5. . . .

       Guide: Conflicts, difficulties with communication, etc.

①   9. *Demonstrate the ability to discern, within one or two interviews, the patient's family's or community worker's reason for referral, the patient's previous psychiatric contacts, knowledge of the family and the community support structure, and the necessary mental status information to construct a formulation and tentative diagnosis.*

10. *Be able to demonstrate a knowledge of and an ability to use appropriately a variety of interviewing techniques:*
    10.1. *Adults*
    10.2. *Children (use of play materials)*
    10.3. *Families*
    10.4. . . .
    10.5. . . .
11. . . .
12. . . .

B. Assessment in Psychiatry

TERMINAL OBJECTIVE

To be able to perform a competent psychiatric assessment of children, adults, families, and groups.

Guide:
1. Be able to evaluate children, demonstrating skills in applying interviewing techniques that are adapted to the developmental level of the child.
2. Expertise with assessment of children and with adults is expected to merge within the framework of family interview skills.

ENABLING OBJECTIVES

1. *For a minimum of each major category of the most recent edition of either ICD or the DSM classification of diseases, be able to demonstrate, with clinical cases, adults and children, an ability to objectively:*
① 1.1. *Do a competent interview (see Section VIII.A above) of the patient and, where applicable, the patient's family.*
① 1.2. *Collect sufficient data to be able to do a complete diagnostic formulation (see Section VII.C, objective 7) and begin treatment of the patient, the patient's children, and the patient's family. . .*

   Guide: Include data collection from:
   a. The patient
   b. The patient's social system, including family, school, work, and other professionals
   . . . and be able to collate material gained from all these sources into a logical format (see Section VIII.A, objective 1, and Section XVI.C, objective 3) with a clear separation of data from opinion.
① 1.3. *Do a complete mental status examination.*

   Guide: Include:
   1.3.1. General observations of appearance and behavior, e.g., dress, posture, attitude, relationship to examiner, mood, and activity
   1.3.2. Mental activity

1.3.3. Emotional state, as reflected in:
    a. Observation by interviewer
    b. Description by the patient
1.3.4. More specifically:
    a. *Be able to operationally define each of the following items.*
    b. *Be able to order your findings under logical groups such as:*
        1.3.4.1. *THINKING*
            Thought Functions
            Ability to learn and retain information
            Attention
            Concentration
            Insight and understanding
            Memory, recent and remote
            Orientation: time, place, and person
            All factors tested by standard intelligence tests
            . . .
            . . .

            Thought Form
            General:
               Attitude
            Specific:
               Ambivalent thinking
               Autistic thinking
               Circumstantiality
               Clang associations
               Flight of ideas
               Loose associations
               Neologism formation
               Stereotype
               Tangential thinking
               Word salad
               . . .
               . . .

            Perceptual Disturbances:
               Delusions
               Depersonalization
               Derealization
               Hallucinations
               . . .
               . . .

            Thought Content
            Suicidal and homocidal ideation
            Grandiose ideation
            Obsessions
            Phobias
            Preoccupations

Ruminations

. . .

. . .

Thought Flow
Increase. decrease

. . .

. . .

1.3.4.2. *FEELING*
Anxiety
Depression
Elation
Flat affect
Fluctuations in affect
Inappropriate affect

. . .

. . .

1.3.4.3. *BEHAVIOR*
Verbal
Nonverbal
  Static:
   . Dress
    Posture
    Grooming
  Dynamic:
    Vocal—tone, inflection, rate, cadence, loud-
      ness
    Motor—facial expressions
    Observed —activity level, type of activity
    Reported (probably not strictly in mental
      status recording)
1.3.4.4. Congruity of thinking, feeling, and behavior
1.3.4.5. Motivation
1.3.4.6. . . .
1.3.4.7. . . .

1.3.5. . . .
1.3.6. . . .

②   **1.4.** *Do a complete physical (including full neurological) examination (and also demonstrate an awareness of some of the positive/negative effects of so doing).*

②   **1.5.** *Construct a problem list with realistic goals and degree of attainment criteria set for each problem or grouping of problems.*

①   **1.6.** *State a formulation (see Section VII.C, objective 7, and Section VII.A, objective 4) (and assess dangerousness to self and others).*

①   **1.7.** *State a differential diagnosis.*

①   **1.8.** *State the provisional diagnosis.*

      1.9. *State necessary steps for future investigations that would lead to:*

①   *1.9.1. Definitive diagnosis*

①   *1.9.2. Treatment categories*
①   *1.9.3. A prognostic statement*

2. *Be able to classify the following psychological tests under the headings* objective *and* projective:

②   *2.1.*   *Bender Gestalt*
④   *2.2.*   *Blacky Pictures*
③   *2.3.*   *Children's Apperception Test (CAT)*
④   *2.4.*   *Denver Developmental Scale*
④   *2.5.*   *Eysenck Personality Inventory*
③   *2.6.*   *Gesell Developmental Scale*
③   *2.7.*   *House—Tree—Person*
④   *2.8.*   *Illinois Test of Psycholinguistic Abilities (ITPA)*
③   *2.9.*   *MMPI (Minnesota Multiphasic Personality Inventory)*
④Ⓐ③Ⓐ   *2.10.*   *Raven's Progressive Matrixes*
④   *2.11.*   *Reitan Battery*
③   *2.12.*   *Rorschach Ink Blot Test*
④   *2.13.*   *16 PF (Personality Factor)*
③   *2.14.*   *Stanford–Binet*
③   *2.15.*   *Thematic Apperception Test (TAT)*
③   *2.16.*   *Vineland Social Maturity Scale*
②   *2.17.*   *WAIS (Wechsler Adult Intelligence Scale)*
②   *2.18.*   *WISC (Wechsler Intelligence Scale for Children)*
       2.19. . . .
       2.20. . . .
       and be able to state for each of these tests:

②   a. *Indications for use*
③   b. *Structure of test (including major subtests)*
④   c. *Standardization*
③   d. *Objectivity*
③   e. *Reliability*
③   f. *Validity (face, content, construct, concurrent, predictive)*
③   g. *Effect on performance of: sex, IQ, physical handicaps, medications, test situation variables, psychological meaning to subject being tested, social and cultural background, and so on.*

②   3. *Be able to utilize positive and negative laboratory test results in formulating clinical cases.*

      Guide:
      N.B.: See Section XIII, objectives 5.3–5.6.
      See Section IV.C.i, objective 3.
      See Section III.G, objective 1.

    4. *Be able to demonstrate an ability to conduct an assessment of a family (see Section XVI.C, objective 3).*

    5. *Be able to state and critically review the indications, contraindications, and procedure for assessments using short-acting barbiturates.*

Guide:
5.1. As a diagnostic aid:
Catatonia from depressive stupor
Organic from functional
5.2. As a means of collecting data
6. *Be able to present all the data gleaned in objectives 1–5 above:*
    6.1. *In written form as a well-organized, easy-to-access case summary*
    6.2. *In verbal form as a succinct, relevant, accurate summary of the findings*
    6.3. *In a manner that can be easily understood by both the patient and professionals (all disciplines)*
7. . . .
8. . . .

C. Nosology

TERMINAL OBJECTIVE

To understand the rationale behind the use of nosology and to apply practically the nosology (DSM or ICD) in use at present.

ENABLING OBJECTIVES

③ 1. *Be able to discuss briefly the historical development of psychiatric nosology.*

Guide: Include the work of:
1.1. Charcot, J.   DSM I
1.2. Kraepelin, E.   DSM II
1.3. Freud, S.   ICD
1.4. APA   DSM III
1.5. International
       committee   ICD 9
1.6. . . .
1.7. . . .

② 2. *Be able to list and define the headings and subheadings of a current classification manual, e.g., DSM, ICD.*

③ 3. *Be able to list the purposes of nosology.*

Guide: Include:
3.1. The development of a common professional language
3.2. As a guide to therapy and prognosis
3.3. To shape the direction of research and theory
3.4. . . .
3.5. . . .

② 4. *Be able to discuss the psychiatric limitations of current classifications.*
     5. . . .
     6. . . .

Section IX.　Psychiatric Emergencies and Reactive Disorders

GENERAL PLAN

A. Crisis Theory
B. Psychiatric Emergencies
C. Suicide
D. Transient Situational and Reactive Disorders
　i. Stress Reaction
　ii. Acute Grief Reaction
　iii. Combat Neuroses
　iv. Acute Culture-Bound Reactions

A. Crisis Theory*

TERMINAL OBJECTIVE

　　To be able to accurately assess and make an appropriate therapeutic response to a clinical case in a crisis reaction.

Guide: For the purposes of this section, a crisis may be defined as a disruption of homeostasis and adaptation caused by a threat to the individual, whether exogenous or endogenous, in which the individual's usual problem-solving techniques do not work.

ENABLING OBJECTIVES

　　1. Given the appropriate life history of a presenting crisis reaction, be able to assess and describe:

①⑦①⚠　　*1.1. The repetitive (characterological) behavior (coping) patterns that the patient exhibits under stress*

②　　*1.2. The historical origin of such behavior patterns where the origin can be identified.*

③　　*1.3. The manner in which the patient perceives the precipitating events and the influence of self concept on distorting perception where this is applicable*

②　　*1.4. The problem-solving ability of the patient*

③　　*1.5. The ease with which the patient is capable of broadening his coping repertoire (alternative modes of coping)*

①　　*1.6. The resources available to help the patient (e.g., significant others)*

　　1.7. . . .

　　1.8. . . .

　　2. Be able to demonstrate a working knowledge of other principles and uses of crisis theory, including:

②　　*2.1. The concept of habitual problem-solving responses*

---

*Although not reaching a .01 level of significance, there was a definite trend in this section for Australians to assign the objectives a lower priority rank than the Americans or Canadians.

ⓐ   *2.2. Crisis as a cause of personal and social disequilibrium*
ⓐ   *2.3. Common characteristics of crisis reactions*
ⓑ   *2.4. Usual duration of crisis reactions*
ⓐ   *2.5. The implications of therapy with the fact that resolution of crisis*
        may be adaptive or maladaptive
ⓐ   *2.6. Recent advances in treatment approaches using crisis theory and*
        crisis intervention
ⓐ   *2.7. The implications of crisis theory for psychotherapy*
        2.8. . . .
        2.9. . . .
ⓑ   *3. Be able to state briefly the physical and emotional and cognitive re-*
     sponses in the preimpact and postimpact stages of crisis
     4. . . .
     5. . . .

B. Psychiatric Emergencies

TERMINAL OBJECTIVE

To be able to identify, assess, and manage any urgent psychiatric condition, whether functional or organic, that compels a person to seek immediate treatment or that impels significant others to seek such treatment for the person, and where immediate treatment would contribute to the likelihood of the patient's recovery or provide urgently needed protection.

ENABLING OBJECTIVES

ⓐ   *1. Be able to identify, assess, and manage psychiatric emergencies.*

Guide: Among emergencies that might be included are:
1.1. Acute affective states
1.2. Acute paranoid states
1.3. Acute schizophrenic states
1.4. Anxiety and panic
1.5. Assaultive states
1.6. Delirium
1.7. Emergencies in children and adolescents
1.8. Epileptic attacks
1.9. Fugues and disassociative states
1.10. Homicide
1.11. Intoxications
1.12. Metabolic disorders of the CNS
1.13. Psychosocial disintegration
1.14. Suicidal behavior (see Topic C below)
1.15. Self mutilation
1.16. . . .
1.17. . . .

2. . . .
3. . . .

C. Suicide

TERMINAL OBJECTIVE

To be capable of identifying, assessing, and managing patients who have made a suicide attempt and patients who are potentially suicidal.

ENABLING OBJECTIVES

①   *1. Be able to define suicide, parasuicide, and attempted suicide.*
      2. Be able to state, for the subjects of suicide and attempted suicide:
②   *2.1. Epidemiological data*
②   *2.1.1. Rate*
②   *2.1.2. Influence of age, sex, and socioeconomic and marital status*
③   *2.1.3. Religion*
②   *2.1.4. Pathology*
③   *2.1.5. Other factors*
②   *2.2. Timing*
③   *2.2.1. Time of day, of year*
③   *2.2.2. Relation to anniversary dates*
          2.2.3. . . .
          2.2.4. . . .
②   *2.3. Frequently encountered biological, psychological, and sociocultural components of contributing, precipitating, and "state-sustaining" factors*
       2.4. . . .
       2.5. . . .
③   *3. Be able to state several common characteristics of those cases that can be grouped under each section of any major classification schema.*

       Guide:
       3.1. "Intrapersonal" suicide, "interpersonal" suicide, and "logical" suicide
       3.2. Be able to give the implications for management of your method of classifying suicidal patients.
       3.3. . . .
       3.4. . . .

①   *4. Be able to state factors that impair ego control and thus increase the risk of suicide in susceptible individuals.*
①   *5. Be able to list three common warning signs that can be elicited in an interview with a potentially suicidal patient.*
①   *6. Be able to relate known psychopathology to the potential for suicide, and be able to discuss the limitations on the ability to estimate suicidal potential in each case.*

③   7. *Be able to give an account of a minimum of one major suicide preven-*
       tion program, noting in particular the validity of the research design
       used to assess its success or failure.
②   8. *Be able to list characteristics that help one clinically differentiate pa-*
       tients whose attempts to commit suicide have a reasonable probability
       of being unsuccessful from those who have a high probability of success
       if a suicidal act is carried out.
       9. *Demonstrate an ability to assess and treat potentially suicidal patients.*
      10. *. . .*
      11. *. . .*

D. Transient Situational and Reactive Disorders

TERMINAL OBJECTIVE

   To be able to differentiate and manage appropriately those aspects of
a patient's presenting problems that represent transient situational
phenomena.

i. Stress Reaction (Including Posttraumatic and Adjustment Disorders)

ENABLING OBJECTIVES

①   1. *Be able to state, for any given clinical example, factors that affect adjust-*
       ment to acute stress.

       Guide:
       1.1. Prestress personality
       1.2. Physical factors—nutrition, infection, injury, exposure
       1.3. Personal resources coping repertoire (cognitive and emotional),
            problem-solving ability
       1.4. Interpersonal resources
       1.5. Social resources
       1.6. . . .
       1.7. . . .
③   2. *Be able to give a clinical description of a stress reaction, clearly separat-*
       ing the phases of the reaction:

       Guide:
       2.1. Threat (preimpact)
       2.2. Impact
       2.3. Recoil
       2.4. Posttraumatic (postimpact)
③   3. *Be able to demonstrate familiarity with the following aspects of manage-*
       ment:
③   3.1. *Leadership role*

②   *3.2. Crisis therapy*
③   *3.3. Posttraumatic support*
       3.4. . . .
       3.5. . . .
    4. . . .
    5. . . .

ii. Acute Grief Reaction

ENABLING OBJECTIVES

1. Be able to demonstrate an ability to assess, accurately diagnose, and manage:
①   *1.1. Normal grief responses*
①   *1.2. Stress-specific responses, such as acute grief, chronic grief, and inhibited grief*
②   *1.3. Nonspecific mixed responses*
       1.4. . . .
       1.5. . . .
①   *2. Be able to do or supervise, or both, short-term interventions and management of pathological responses to loss.*
③   *3. Be able to state the probable outcome for each of the conditions listed in objective 1 above both with and without intervention.*
    4. . . .
    5. . . .

iii. Combat Neuroses

ENABLING OBJECTIVES

①   *1. Be able to list and discuss predisposing factors.*

     Guide:
     1.1. Age
     1.2. Civil status
     1.3. Education
     1.4. Premorbid personality
     1.5. . . .
     1.6. . . .
③   *2. Be able to accurately assess the clinical features, form a management plan, and relate factors such as compensation and premorbid personality to the prognosis.*
    3. . . .
    4. . . .

iv. Acute Culture-Bound Reactions*

ENABLING OBJECTIVES

1. *Be able to state for acute culture-bound syndromes the:*
   ④   *1.1. Clinical features*
   ④   *1.2. Epidemiology*
   ④   *1.3. Management and prognosis*

      Guide:
      a. Amok
      b. Koro
      c. Latah
      1.4. . . .
      1.5. . . .
2. *. . .*
3. *. . .*

Section X.   Psyche and Soma and Liaison Psychiatry

TERMINAL OBJECTIVES

1. To be able to recognize patients with psychophysiological disorders and psychosocial reactions to physical illness in terms of symptoms, signs, and differential diagnosis.
2. To have the required awareness and knowledge of multifactorial etiology and the important interactions between biological (neuroanatomical, physiological, and biochemical) and psychosocial factors in the production of bodily malfunction and psychosocial sequelae of physical illness.
3. To be able to prescribe treatments, including education of the patient, and to be able to support your choice of treatment by reference to recent research findings.

ENABLING OBJECTIVES

①   *1. Be able to discuss current conceptual understandings of the interaction of psyche and soma and to list examples of the disorders arising therefrom using either the DSM or the ICD classification scheme.*
    2. Be able to discuss the interaction of psyche and soma from biological, psychological, and sociological points of view, including:
②   *2.1. Biological: Be able to describe the neuroanatomical, physiological, biochemical, and endocrine bases of psychological factors in physical illness. Include:*
       2.1.1. Limbic system
       2.1.2. Hypothalamus

*See Section V.A for more details.

         2.1.3. Autonomic nervous system

         2.1.4. Endocrine system

②   *2.2. Psychological: Be able to describe recent developments and theoretical constructs from learning theory (include biofeedback) and personality theory (include psychodynamics) relevant to the initiation, exacerbation, or continuation of a physical disorder.*

②   *2.3. Sociological: Be able to discuss the role of environmental changes and life events in inducing stress that may lead to the initiation, exacerbation, or continuation of a physical disorder.*

        Guide: Holmes and Rahe, Life Change Units

②   *2.4. Reaction to illness: Be able to state the major tenets of theories relevant to psychosocial reactions to physical and emotional illness.*

    2.5. . . .

    2.6. . . .

  3. Be able to state the basic principles of diagnosis, formulation, and differential diagnosis in "liaison" psychiatry.

    3.1. For those conditions for which liaison consultation is frequently requested, including:

        3.1.1. Disorders without demonstrable organic findings but that "suggest" physical illness:

            3.1.1.1. Involuntary

            Guide:

            Examples: Briquet's syndrome, conversion, psychalgia

            3.1.1.2. Voluntary without apparent goal

            Guide:

            Example: Factitious disorders such as Munchausen's syndrome

            3.1.1.3. Voluntary with an apparent goal

            Guide:

            Example: Malingering

        3.1.2. Depression

        3.1.3. Psychological factors in physical conditions

        3.1.4. Psychotic reactions:

            3.1.4.1. Postoperative

            3.1.4.2. Postpartum

            3.1.4.3. . . .

            3.1.4.4. . . .

        3.1.5. Other

            Guide:

            Examples: anorexia nervosa; factitious illness that is self-induced, e.g., dermatitis artefacta; "special" problems of the ICU or the renal dialysis unit

        3.1.6. . . .

        3.1.7. . . .

be able to state:

    a. Definition, ICD or DSM

    b. Occurrence of symptoms and signs in "normal" subjects

    c. Physiological basis

    d. Association with other clinical phenomena

    e. The biopsychosociocultural and environmental components which are important in understanding the predisposing, precipitating, and sustaining factors involved in the illness in question

    f. Clinical features

    g. Common differential diagnostic possibilities

    h. In the hospital setting, techniques for assisting the nursing team to create a psychologically (as well as physically) therapeutic milieu for the patient

3.2. Be able to respond appropriately to the "type" of consultation being requested (see Section XVII.D, objective 2).

① *3.3. Be able, in the clinical setting, to collate knowledge from all the areas in objective 2 above into a diagnostic formulation and to offer a differential diagnosis in any of the disorders in objective 3.1. above. (See also Section VII.C, objective 7.)*

② *3.4. Be able to demonstrate an ability to recognize and assess both the biological and the psychological significance of medical and surgical investigations and treatment.*

① *3.5. Be able, in the role of psychiatric consultant, to recognize psychosocial complications of physical illness and the treatment in addition to indications or contraindications, or both, for the present treatment.*

    Guide:

    3.5.1. Reserpine in hypertension leading to depression

    3.5.2. . . .

    3.5.3. . . .

3.6. . . .

3.7. . . .

  4. Be able to state the basic principles of treatment and prognosis, including:

① *4.1. For disorders in which psychological factors are associated with a physical illness, be able to list indications, contraindications, and prognosis for treatments commonly utilized (e.g., Section XV.B, objective 3).*

① *4.2. Be able to demonstrate, in the clinical setting, an ability to inform patients appropriately of the nature and treatment of the problems listed in objective 4.1 above.*

① *4.3. Be able to accurately apply treatment knowledge in the clinical setting (with particular reference to the application of clinical skills in the general hospital ward).*

4.4. Be able, in the clinical setting, to state the objectives of the chosen treatment modalities and the factors that may be relevant in determining the outcome.

4.5. . . .
4.6. . . .
5. . . .
6. . . .

Section XI.   The Neuroses, Personality Disorders, Addictions, and Sexual Disorders —Including Disorders That Are Associated Primarily with Affective, Anxiety, "Somatoform," Dissociative, Factitious, Impulse-Control, Drug-Use, Psychosexual, and Personality Problems

GENERAL PLAN

A. The Neuroses
B. Personality Disorders
C. Drug-Use Disorders
D. Psychosexual Disorders

TERMINAL OBJECTIVE

On the basis of a broad knowledge of modern theories of etiology and the various treatment modalities and with knowledge of the limitations thereof, to be able to assess, formulate, diagnose, and treat the conditions discussed in this section.

GENERAL ENABLING OBJECTIVES APPLICABLE TO ALL TOPICS

1. Be able to make succinct, relevant, and critical statements (where appropriate) for each of the disorders subsumed under the titles listed above (i.e., ICD or DSM classification) under the following headings:

①   *1.1. Definition (ICD or DSM), incidence, and prevalence*
①   *1.2. Occurrence of symptoms or signs, or both, in "normal" subjects*
②   *1.3. Physiological basis (e.g., neurophysiological, endocrine)*
②   *1.4. Association with other clinical phenomena*
②   *1.5. Predisposing or contributing factors* ⎫   *a. Biological*
                                   ⎪   *b. Psychological*
①   *1.6. Precipitating factors* ⎬   *c. Social*
②   *1.7. Sustaining factors* ⎭   *d. Cultural*
                                            e. Environmental

①   *1.8. Clinical features*

Guide: Include repetitive *patterns* of behavior.

①   *1.9. Differential diagnosis*

①   *1.10. Course with and without treatment*
①   *1.11. Types of treatment most commonly used, the objectives for each*
        type of treatment or combination of treatments, the rationale be-
        hind their use, and their probable effectiveness (noting studies
        that support and refute their postulated efficacy)
②   *1.12. Other factors that are relevant in determining outcome*
③   *1.13. Historical development of the concept*
②   *1.14. Modern theories and hypotheses concerning etiology (see specific*
        objectives following)
       1.15. Aspects of primary prevention
       1.16. Characteristics of high-risk "groups" where appropriate
       1.17. . . .
       1.18. . . .
   2. Be able, using clinical examples, to assess, formulate, and plan the
      management of conditions subsumed under the titles listed above.
   3. . . .
   4. . . .

ENABLING OBJECTIVES APPLICABLE TO SPECIFIC
TOPICS

A. The Neuroses [Including Affective (Intermittent), Anxiety,
   Somatoform, and Dissociative Disorders]

①   *1. Be able to relate the onset of symptoms to a "precipitating" event or*
       events, both intrapsychic and environmental, and present a dynamic
       formulation of the case, taking into account the patient's characterologi-
       cal structure, his present and past stresses, and characteristic coping and
       defense mechanisms.

       Guide:
       See Section VII.C, objective 7
②   *2. Be able to demonstrate a working knowledge of current etiological the-*
       ories; include the ability to discuss important contributions by major
       authors and relate them to presented clinical material.

       Guide: Include:
       2.1. Classical psychoanalytic theories, including the work of Freud,
            Klein, and Jung
       2.2. Neo-Freudian concepts of neuroses, including the work of Sullivan,
            Adler, and Horney
       2.3. Contemporary formulations of "neuroses," including the work of
            Erikson, Engel, and Berne
       2.4. Theories based on learning theory
       2.5. See also Section VII.
       2.6. . . .
       2.7. . . .
①   *3. Be able to demonstrate, with clinical case material, a working knowledge*
       of current treatment modalities.

Guide: Include:

3.1. The symptomatic use of psychotropic drugs in the treatment of these disorders, including contraindications and side effects of these drugs

3.2. The use of appropriate psychotherapeutic measures—individual, family, group, and milieu therapies—in short- or long-term treatment. Be able to discuss possible transference and countertransference issues that might arise in therapy, and set realistic treatment goals for the patient.

3.3. Be able to demonstrate a working knowledge of techniques of behavior therapy applicable to the treatment goals for the patient.

3.4. Be able to determine, in any given case, which of the above treatment modalities, or combinations thereof, is appropriate, and then mobilize whatever treatment resources are necessary.

3.5. . . .

3.6. . . .

④ *4. Be able to describe the significance to modern psychiatric practice of the principal findings and concepts advanced by major authorities not previously referred to in this section.*

Guide: Include:

4.1. Eysenck, H. J.

4.2. Gillespie, R. D., 1929

4.3. Hill, Denis

4.4. Kendall

4.5. Kiloh and Garside, 1963

4.6. Lewis, Aubrey, 1934

4.7. Leighton, A. H. (or comparable epidemiological study)

4.8. Mapother, W., 1926

4.9. Rees, 1961

4.10. Shagass, C., and Jones, 1958

4.11. Stenstedt, 1959

4.12. . . .

4.13. . . .

5. . . .

6. . . .

B. Personality Disorders [Including Affective (Intermittent and Atypical), Factitious, and Impulse-Control Disorders]

② *1. Be able to state the principal tenets of the following theoretical frameworks:*

1.1. Classical psychoanalytic concepts

1.1.1. Freud, S.

1.1.2. Klein, M.

1.1.3. Winnicott, D. W.

1.1.4. . . .

1.1.5. . . .

③   *1.2. Separation and attachment studies*
           1.2.1. Bowlby, J.
           1.2.2. Spitz, R. A.
           1.2.3. . . .
           1.2.4. . . .
③   *1.3. Follow-up of studies of childhood antecedents*
           1.3.1. Robins, L. N.
           1.3.2. . . .
           1.3.3. . . .
③   *1.4. Ethological studies*
           1.4.1. Harlow, H. F.
           1.4.2. . . .
           1.4.3. . . .
        1.5. . . .
        1.6. . . .
     2. Describe the following treatment approaches:
②   *2.1. Symptomatic use of drugs*
①   *2.2. Use of appropriate psychotherapeutic measures*
②   *2.2.1. Group and milieu therapy*
①   *2.2.2. Short- and long-term treatment of personality disorders*
            2.2.3. . . .
            2.2.4. . . .
②   *2.3. Behavior therapy*
②   *2.3.1. Reinforcement techniques for appropriate and adaptive*
               behaviors
            2.3.2. . . .
            2.3.3. . . .
        2.4. . . .
        2.5. . . .
①   *3. Be able to set realistic goals with and for the patient.*
④   *4. Be able to describe the significance to modern psychiatric practice of*
        the principal findings and concepts of major contributors to our knowl-
        edge of the personality disorders.

        Guide:
        4.1. Cleckley, H.
        4.2. Glueck, S.
        4.3. Guze, S. B.
        4.4. Lombroso, C.
        4.5. Pinel, P.
        4.6. Robins, L. N.
        4.7. Sheldon, W. H.
        4.8. . . .
        4.9. . . .
     5. . . .
     6. . . .

C. Drug-Use Disorders (Including Alcoholism and Drug Dependencies)

③ 1. *Be able to discuss current issues related to alcoholism and drug dependencies, including:*
    1.1. *Historical background*
    1.2. *Prevalent community attitudes and legislation*
    1.3. *Current definitions*
    1.4. *Recent community studies*
    1.5. *Research*
    1.6. . . .
    1.7. . . .

① 2. *Be able to describe signs and symptoms and identify, in the clinical setting, acute and chronic intoxication and abstinence phenomena.*

    Guide: Include each of the substances noted in the ICD or DSM classification of diseases.

② 3. *Be able to give examples of pertinent pharmacological facts related to the drug.*

② 4. *Be able to state the interactions of sociological, personality, pharmacological, and conditioning factors in various phases of the habituation process.*

② 5. *Be able to demonstrate, with clinical case material, the ability to diagnose and treat, without prejudice, abstinence syndromes and to manage the patient's ongoing therapeutic program (including use of Antabuse with alcoholics).*

    Guide:
    5.1. Alcohol
    5.2. The opioids
    5.3. Barbiturates
    5.4. Meprobamate
    5.5. . . .
    5.6. . . .

6. *Be able to list biochemical tests for substances noted in the ICD or DSM classification of diseases (see Section XIII, objective 5.5.2).*

7. *With respect to each of the drug-use disorders and for the following treatment approaches:*
    7.1. *Group support, e.g., Alcoholics Anonymous*
    7.2. *Therapeutic community*
    7.3. *Behavior modification*
    7.4. *Psychotherapy*
    7.5. *Psychopharmacology, e.g., disulfiram, methadone*
    7.6. . . .
    7.7. . . .
    be able to state:
    a. *Indications*
    b. *Contraindications where applicable*

  c. *Incompatibility with other approaches*
  d. *Side and toxic effects where applicable*
  e. *Efficacy and factors governing "limitations" of the method*
  f. *Method for administration of the treatment*
  g. *. . .*
  h. *. . .*

  Guide:
  This is in addition to Topic A, objective 3, above.
  8. *. . .*
  9. *. . .*

D. Psychosexual Disorders

① 1. *Be able to relate onset and recurrences of pathological deviant behavior to predisposing and precipitating factors, and important life conflicts in the individual.*

② 2. *Be able to discuss various treatment approaches commonly used in the management of the psychosexual disorders.*

  Guide: This discussion should include:
  2.1. Psychotherapy, particularly individual and group therapy
  2.2. Behavior therapy, particularly aversive techniques
  2.3. Use of physical methods. including hormone therapy
  2.4. The techniques popularized by Masters and Johnson
  2.5. . . .
  2.6. . . .
  3. *. . .*
  4. *. . .*

Section XII.   The "Functional" Psychoses

GENERAL PLAN

① A. The Schizophrenic Disorders

  Guide: Include:
  1. Simple type
  2. Hebephrenic type
  3. Catatonic type
  4. Paranoid type
  5. Acute schizophrenic episode
  6. "Latent" schizophrenia
  7. Residual schizophrenia or defect state
  8. Schizoaffective (manic and depressed types)
  9. Childhood schizophrenia
  10. Others. including mixed or undifferentiated

①   B. Paranoid Disorders

      Guide:
      1. Paranoia
      2. Shared (folie à deux)
      3. Others, including involutional paraphrenia

①   C. Affective Disorders—Psychotic

      Guide:
      1. Single or recurrent manic episodes
      2. Single or recurrent depressive episodes, including involutional melancholia
      3. Bipolar or circular

②   D. "Borderline" States

       E. Brief Reactive Disorders

③   F. Atypical "Psychoses"

       G. Other Psychoses

TERMINAL OBJECTIVES

1. To know about, and be able to communicate clearly on, classification, etiology, clinical features, differential diagnosis, specific treatments, general management, and prognosis of the functional psychoses.
2. To be able to interview, diagnose, and manage the treatment of patients suffering from the functional psychoses.

ENABLING OBJECTIVES APPLICABLE TO ALL FUNCTIONAL PSYCHOSES: GENERAL

     1. Be able to demonstrate an understanding of the historical evolution of present-day concepts of the term "psychosis" and the group of conditions known as the functional psychoses by being able to give an account of:

④   *1.1. The contributions made by important historical figures*

       Guide:
       1.1.1. Bleuler, E.
       1.1.2. Hecker, E.
       1.1.3. Kraepelin, E.
       1.1.4. Kahlbaum, K. L.
       1.1.5. . . .
       1.1.6. . . .

④   *1.2. The views about the functional psychoses that prevailed at differing points in time*

①   *1.3. Present-day views about the concept of schizophrenia*

①   *1.4. The classification of the affective disorders*

③   *1.5. The validity of claims made for the nosological independence of certain atypical and other psychoses*

      1.6. ...

      1.7. ...

2. *Be able to demonstrate a knowledge of the etiological hypotheses by knowing the more important cause–effect relationships that have been postulated for the functional psychoses, and the body of empirical knowledge that is adduced to support each of them.*

①   *2.1. Biological (including genetic)*

①   *2.2. Psychological*

①   *2.3. Social*

①   *2.4. Cultural*

②   *2.5. Other combinations*

      2.6. ...

      2.7. ...

3. *Be able to state the following characteristics of each of the functional psychoses (in detail for Topics A–D, briefly for E–G):*

②   *3.1. Distribution of the disorder in the population*

③   *3.1.1. Prevalence, incidence, characteristics of affected persons*

③   *3.1.2. Places, times, and all other epidemiological features*

③▽②△   *3.1.3. Description of at least one major epidemiological study*

           3.1.4. ...

           3.1.5. ...

②   *3.2. Established physical characteristics*

②   *3.2.1. Biochemical*

②   *3.2.2. Physiological*

③   *3.2.3. EEG*

③   *3.2.4. Body build*

           3.2.5. ...

           3.2.6. ...

①   *3.3. Symptoms and signs of each condition*

②   *3.3.1. Difference between disorders of expression and experience (phenomenological)*

①   *3.3.2. Symptoms that are of high diagnostic value by their presence or absence*

②   *3.3.3. Symptoms characteristically found when the psychosis is mild or severe, and in early or late stages*

           3.3.4. ...

           3.3.5. ...

③   *3.4. The psychological tests that are employed in diagnosis and the results that typify the specific psychosis*

②   *3.5. Natural history of the condition*

③   *3.5.1. Any cultural, social, or secular differences and changes that have occurred with the development of modern treatment*

           3.5.2. ...

           3.5.3. ...

②   *3.6. Associations of each with other clinical phenomena (if applicable)*

      3.7. ...

      3.8. ...

②   4. *Be able to list, compare, and contrast the categories used to classify the psychoses in the DSM III and the ICDA classification schemes.*

      5. *Be able to demonstrate comprehensive knowledge of the following factors for each therapeutic modality used in the treatment of each of the major psychoses:*

①   5.1. *Indications*

①   5.2. *Contraindications*

①   5.3. *Side effects (toxic effects where applicable)*

①   5.4. *Technique of its application*

①   5.5. *Mechanism of action (biological, psychological, social)*

①   5.6. *Objectives for each type of treatment or combination of treatments and their probable effectiveness (noting studies that support and refute their postulated efficacy)*

      5.7. *Other factors that are relevant to determining outcome*

②   6. *Be able to specify the value and the role of other members of the health care team in the treatment of psychoses.*

①   7. *Be able to list the major prognostic indicators.*

②   8. *Be able to discuss the means by which the psychosis might possibly be prevented.*

      9. . . .

      10. . . .

ENABLING OBJECTIVES APPLICABLE TO ALL FUNCTIONAL PSYCHOSES: CLINICAL

      1. *Be able to demonstrate, by conducting clinical interviews with patients suffering from major psychoses, the capacity to:*

①   1.1. *Establish a therapeutic relationship.*

①   1.2. *Elicit a history and conduct a mental examination.*

①   1.3. *Produce a formulation of the case, including:*

①   1.3.1. *The differential diagnosis with the reasons*

①   1.3.2. *All the possible etiological factors together with their possible modes of interaction*
                Guide: Predisposing, precipitating, and sustaining factors — biological, psychological, social, cultural, and environmental aspects

①   1.3.3. *The prognosis and plan of management*

②   1.3.4. *See Section VIII.B, objective 1.5, and Section VII.C, objective 7.*

      1.3.5. . . .

      1.3.6. . . .

      1.4. *Plan the management of the case, including:*

①   1.4.1. *Further investigations such as psychological tests to resolve diagnostic problems*

①   1.4.2. *A treatment program tailored to the individual patient with techniques for the prevention of a relapse once a remission has been achieved*

1.4.3. . . .
1.4.4. . . .
1.5. . . .
1.6. . . .
2. . . .
3. . . .

ENABLING OBJECTIVES APPLICABLE TO SPECIFIC FUNCTIONAL PSYCHOSES

A. The Schizophrenic Disorders

①   General and clinical enabling objectives as above.

B. Paranoid Disorders

③   *1. Be able to draw a flow diagram to indicate the development of paranoia.*

   Guide: Proceed from:
   1.1. The preliminary threat
   1.2. Onset
   1.3. Early phase
   1.4. Preliminary focus
   1.5. The pseudocommunity
②   *2. Be able to draw up three lists, side by side, comparing and contrasting the clinical features of paranoia, paranoid schizophrenia, and paranoid states secondary to organic cerebral syndromes.*
   3. . . .
   4. . . .

C. Affective Disorders—Psychotic

①   *1. Be able to discuss the nature of the relationship between suicide and affective disorders.*
①   *2. Be able to state features of the examination of the patient necessary to detect suicidal intent.*
②   *3. Be able to discuss both the theoretical and the clinical usefulness of the basis for unipolar–bipolar classification.*
   4. . . .
   5. . . .

D. "Borderline" States

②   *1. Define borderline states and describe other similar concepts such as "pseudoneurotic schizophrenia," "ambulatory schizophrenia," and "as if states," together with their relationship to schizophrenia. (Note: Classified as Personality disorder DSM III.)*

② 2. *List the clinical features of borderline states.*

    Guide: Include:

    2.1. Patient's relationship to himself

    2.2. Patient's relationship to others

    2.3. Patient's relationship to work

    2.4. Affect (pananxiety)

    2.5. Impulsivity and aggression

    2.6. Self concept, self context

    2.7. . . .

    2.8. . . .

3. . . .

4. . . .

E. Brief Reactive Disorders

1. *Be able to operationally define the term "reactive" psychosis.*
2. *Be able to list and describe those disorders that could be considered "reactive" using both the ICD A and DSM III classification schemes.*
3. . . .
4. . . .

F. Atypical "Psychoses"

1. *Be able to list and give a brief "operational" definition of each of the proposed subtypes of the atypical psychoses.*

    Guide:

    1.1. Unusual variants of the major psychoses

③   1.1.1. "Mixed states"—affective (Kraepelin, E.)

③   1.1.1.1. Manic stupor

③   1.1.1.2. Depression with psychomotor acceleration

④   1.1.1.3. Other rare combinations, Kraepelin's triad

④   1.1.2. Oneiroid states (oneirophrenia)

④   1.1.3. Pfropfschizophrenia

③   1.1.4. Pseudoneurotic psychoses

        1.1.5. . . .

        1.1.6. . . .

    1.2. Atypical psychoses, which may be valid clinical entities distinct from the major psychoses

④   1.2.1. Cycloid psychoses (Leonhard, K.)

④   1.2.1.1. Anxiety–elation psychosis

④   1.2.1.2. Confusion psychosis

④   1.2.1.3. Motility psychosis

④   1.2.2. Nonsystematic schizophrenias

④   1.2.2.1. Affect-laden paraphrenia

④   1.2.2.2. Schizophrenia

④   1.2.2.3. Periodic catatonia

          1.2.3. . . .
          1.2.4. . . .
    1.3. . . .
    1.4. . . .

2. *Be able to marshal the arguments for and against the hypotheses that schizoaffective disorders are:*

③   *2.1. Minor deviations from the characteristic clinical picture of either schizophrenia or "manic–depressive" psychosis, and are thus of little nosological significance*

③   *2.2. Concurrent manifestations of "manic–depressive" psychosis and schizophrenia in the same individual at the same time.*

③   *2.3. Specific nosological entities*
      2.4. . . .
      2.5. . . .

④ 3. *Be able to describe briefly Gjessing's work on periodic catatonia, with special emphasis on its historical significance.*

    4. *Be able to identify clinically and know how to resolve the diagnostic difficulties presented by:*

④   *4.1. Pfropfschizophrenia (mental retardation)*
④   *4.2. Oneirophrenia (clouding of consciousness)*
      4.3. . . .
      4.4. . . .

    5. . . .
    6. . . .

G. Other Psychoses

1. *Be able to list and give a brief "operational" definition of each of the major proposed subtypes of "other" psychoses.*

    Guide:
    1.1. Known etiology, but closely resembling functional psychoses
①   1.1.1. Symptomatic "schizophrenias"
①   1.1.1.1. Amphetamine psychosis
①   1.1.1.2. Chronic psychosis of temporal lobe epilepsy
②   1.1.1.3. Other organic states, i.e., related to concentration of vitamin B_{12}, folic acid, etc.
③   1.1.1.4. Psychogenic "schizophrenia," schizophreniform psychosis (Langfeldt), benign schizophrenia
            1.1.1.5. . . .
            1.1.1.6. . . .
②   1.1.2. Experimental psychosis
③   1.1.2.1. Drugs
③   1.1.2.2. Sensory deprivation
            1.1.2.3. . . .
            1.1.2.4. . . .
        1.1.3. . . .
        1.1.4. . . .

1.2. Unusual syndromes, some of which can arise by themselves or in the course of a major functional psychosis
④ 1.2.1. Capgras's syndrome
④ 1.2.2. Clerambault's syndrome (erotomania)
④ 1.2.3. Cotard's syndrome (delire de negation)
④ 1.2.4. Othello syndrome (delusional jealousy)
③ 1.2.5. Gilles de la Tourette's syndrome
1.2.6. . . .
1.2.7. . . .
1.3. Psychoses associated with childbearing
② 1.3.1. Psychoses of pregnancy
② 1.3.2. Puerperal psychoses
③ 1.3.3. Lactation psychoses
1.3.4. . . .
1 3.5. . . .
1.4. Psychotic syndromes that have been observed predominantly in certain cultural settings
④ 1.4.1. Amok
④ 1.4.2. Koro
④ 1.4.3. Latah
④ 1.4.4. Piblokto
④ 1.4.5. Windigo
④ 1.4.6. Voodoo
1.4.7. . . .
1.4.8. . . .
1.5. Syndromes that are probably psychogenic, and are sometimes described as "pseudopsychotic"
③ 1.5.1. Hysterical psychosis
③ 1.5.2. Pseudodementia (ganser)
③ 1.5.3. Munchausen's syndrome
③ 1.5.4. Folie à deux, à trois, en masse
1.5.5. . . .
1.5.6. . . .
1.6. . . .
1.7. . . .
③ 2. *Be able to discuss the nosological positions of the "other" psychoses in the light of various etiological theories about them.*

Guide: The relationship of "other" psychoses to:
2.1. The classical functional psychoses
2.2. Organic psychosyndromes
2.3. The neuroses
2.4. . . .
2.5. . . .
③ 3. *For the psychoses related to childbearing, be able to:*
3.1. Differentiate them from psychogenic reactions.
3.2. Assess prognosis.
3.3. Describe the management of several conditions.

    3.4. . . .

    3.5. . . .

③   *4. Be able to discuss the research implications of the "experimental" psychoses, including:*

        4.1. Implications for our understanding of the classical functional psychoses

        4.2. The scope of this research

        4.3. The limitations of this research

        4.4. . . .

        4.5. . . .

④   *5. Be able to discuss the etiological factors of culture-bound psychosyndromes and discuss their nosology in terms of comparative psychiatry.*

    6. . . .

    7. . . .

Section XIII. The Organic Mental Disorders

TERMINAL OBJECTIVE

To be able to recognize the clinical syndromes that can arise from organic disturbance of brain function; have sufficient knowledge of neuroanatomy, physiology, and pathology to appreciate the factors underlying such states; and know the common physical conditions that may produce such states and be able to diagnose and treat them.

ENABLING OBJECTIVES

①   *1. Be able to describe the normal aging process and discuss the effects that aging has on mental functioning.*

    2. Be able to discuss the kinds of mental changes produced by coarse brain disease, including such variables as:

③▽②△*   *2.1. The speed of action of the morbid process*

③†   *2.2. The extent and severity of the brain damage*

③†   *2.3. The duration of the brain damage*

③†   *2.4. The presence of focal lesions*

③†   *2.5. The individual's predisposition*

③   *2.6. The environmental situation*

    2.7. . . .

    2.8. . . .

    3. Be able to describe the symptoms and signs of organic states that may be reversible.

---

*At .008 level of significance.

†At .02 level of significance each of these has priority rankings ▽②△ .

Guide - Use DSM or ICDA classification, but include all the following phenomena:

①   3.1. Delirious states—acute and subacute
①   3.2. Organic stuporous states - apathetic confusional states
①   3.3. Organic twilight states
②   3.4. Other
③   3.4.1. Emotional hyperaesthetic syndromes
②   3.4.2. Depressive and manic syndromes
②   3.4.3. Organic paranoid states (and organic delusional syndromes)
②   3.4.4. Organic hallucinosis
③   3.4.5. Exogenous paranoid hallucinatory syndrome
③   3.4.6. Expansive confabulatory syndrome
②   3.4.7. Amnestic syndromes
          3.4.8. . . .
          3.4.9. . . .

4. *Be able to describe the symptoms and signs of irreversible organic states:*

Guide—Use DSM or ICDA classification, but include all the following phenomena:

①   4.1. Progressive dementia or the chronic brain syndrome
③   4.2. Other
③   4.2.1. Nonprogressive intellectual defect state
③   4.2.2. Chronic emotional hyperaesthetic syndrome
③   4.2.3. Chronic amnestic states
③   4.2.4. Focal syndromes
③   4.2.5. Organic personality syndrome
          4.2.6. . . .
          4.2.7. . . .

5. *Be able to demonstrate the following skills:*

①   5.1. *Perform a thorough clinical examination with emphasis on the nervous system.*

①   5.2. *Conduct a thorough mental status examination with special reference to those tests both neurological and psychological that are used for the assessment of organic mental functioning.*

       Guide: Particular attention should be paid to the use of the WAIS and the Bender-Gestalt tests.

②   5.3. *Recognize the significance of the electroencephalographic abnormalities seen in organic brain disease.*

②   5.4. *State the indications for:*
          5.4.1. *Skull X rays*
          5.4.2. *Lumbar puncture*
          5.4.3. *Brain scan*
          5.4.4. *Cerebral arteriogram*
          5.4.5. *Ventriculogram*
          5.4.6. *Air encephalogram*
          5.4.7. *Echogram*

      5.4.8.   *Computer-assisted axial tomography (EMI or CATscan)*

      5.4.9. . . .

      5.4.10. . . .

  5.5. *State the meaning of deviation from normal values for commonly used hematological and biochemical screening tests.*

      Guide:

      5.5.1. Hematology, enzymes. antibodies. hormones. porphyrins, electrolytes, etc.

      5.5.2. Blood levels of chemotherapeutic agents and "street" drugs

      5.5.3. "Specialized tests," e.g., VDRL. glucose tolerance. creatinine clearance

      5.5.4. . . .

      5.5.5. . . .

②   5.6. *State the meaning of all laboratory findings for the mental health of the patient.*

    5.7. . . .

    5.8. . . .

  6. *For* both *the underlying physical condition* and *the concomitant "psychiatric" organic mental syndrome sequelae in:*

①   6.1.   *Senile dementia*

②*   6.2.   *Cardiovascular disorders—with special attention given to arteriosclerotic dementia*

②*   6.3.   *The presenile dementias—with special attention given to Alzheimer's disease, Pick's disease, Huntington's chorea, Jacob Creutzfeldt's disease, and hepatolenticular degeneration*

②*   6.4.   *Infection of the brain and its coverings—with special attention given to general paresis*

②*   6.5.   *Physical injury to the brain*

②*   6.6.   *Epilepsies*

②*   6.7.   *Cerebral neoplasms, other intracerebral tumors, and conditions causing distortion of cerebral anatomy including hydrocephalus*

①   6.8.   *Toxic states—special attention should be given to alcohol, heavy metals, and commonly used drugs*

②*   6.9.   *Metabolic and biochemical disorders—special attention should be paid to anoxia, hypoglycemia, dehydration, and vitamin deficiencies*

②   6.10. *Demyelinating diseases that affect mental functioning*

    6.11. . . .

    6.12. . . .

    be able, after carrying out the appropriate clinical investigation on a patient, to demonstrate an ability to state and describe the:

①   a. *Etiology*

②   b. *Pathology*

①   c. *Clinical features*

---

*At a .02 to .2 level of significance each of these has priority rankings of ▽①△ .

①   *d. Diagnosis and differential diagnosis*
①   *e. Possible complications and sequelae*
①   *f. Effects of societal expectations in the course of illness*
①   *g. Prognosis with and without intervention*
①   *h. Possible prevention techniques*
      and to initiate:
      i. Treatment and management

     Guide: Objective number 6 can be thought of as a grid.
7. *Be able, in the clinical setting, to differentiate between "pseudodementia"*
   due to depression and chronic brain disease.
8. . . .
9. . . .

Section XIV. The Organic Therapies

GENERAL PLAN

A. Psychopharmacology
B. Convulsive Therapies
C. Psychosurgery
D. Miscellaneous and Little-Used Biological Treatments

A. Psychopharmacology

TERMINAL OBJECTIVE

    To learn about the safe use of psychotropic medications with respect to the prevention and treatment of psychiatric disorders.

ENABLING OBJECTIVES

    1. *Be able to list the major subdivisions of the psychopharmacological agents used in psychiatry under the following headings:*
①   *1.1. Major tranquilizers (neuroleptics)*
①   *1.2. Minor tranquilizers (anxiolytics)*
①   *1.3. Antidepressants*
①   *1.4. Stimulants*
①   *1.5. Anti-Parkinson agents*
①   *1.6. Metallic salts (lithium)*
①   *1.7. Sedative/hypnotics*
②   *1.8. Others (e.g., anticonvulsants, disulfiram)*
①   2. *Be able to list under the groups in objective 1 above the main agents used, by both generic and commercial names.*

    3. Be able to state for each of the groups in objective 1 above:

①   *3.1.*   *Indications*

        Guide: Both for particular type of pharmacotherapy and for the choice of a particular agent

①   *3.2.*   *Contraindications*

        Guide: Biochemical, physiological, psychological

①   *3.3.*   *Incompatibility with other medications (and/or any special diet restrictions), and the mechanism thereof*

        Guide: Absorption, binding, metabolism, excretion

①   *3.4.*   *Drug interaction and effects on clinical lab results*

①   *3.5.*   *Dose, route, timing*

        Guide: Time of day, with respect to meals, etc.

①   *3.6.*   *Side effects and toxic effects*

        Guide: Short-term, long-term

②   *3.7.*   *Theoretical sites of action*

②   *3.8.*   *Theoretical modes of action*

③   *3.9.*   *General chemical formula for the class of drug*

①   *3.10.* *Efficacy*

①   *3.11.* *Prevention and treatment of side and toxic effects*

    3.12. *Time factors*

        Guide:
        a. Length of trial before concluding that therapeutic effect is nil or equivocal
        b. Length of time before trial period without medications is instituted
        c. Use of "drug holidays"

    3.13. *Method for ascertaining whether or not a potentially therapeutic level of medication has been reached in body tissues*

    3.14. *Methods for increasing the likelihood of the patient's continuing to take the prescribed medication on a regular basis*

    3.15. *Factors that influence the quantity of medication you allow the patient to purchase, use of renewals, etc.*

    3.16. . . .

    3.17. . . .

    4. Be able to state and discuss the differences in the use of the drugs listed in objective 1 above from the points of view outlined in objective 3 above between adults and children and "middle" age and psychogeriatric populations.

②   *5. Be able to define and discuss the placebo response (including all non-pharmacological actions of medications).*

    6. Be able to state the relationship between serum or plasma levels of a drug and its clinical efficacy or toxicity, or both, where such relationships are known.

Guide: Include:

6.1. Dilantin

6.2. Lithium

6.3. Tricyclic and tetracyclic antidepressants

6.4. Phenothiazines

6.5. Butyrophenones

6.6. . . .

6.7. . . .

7. *Be able to describe the "interaction" of medication and psychotherapy.*

③ 8. *Be able to describe a research design for investigation of the clinical safety and usefulness of a new chemotherapeutic agent.*

Guide: Include need for double blind, crossover, placebo, etc.

9. . . .

10. . . .

B. Convulsive Therapies

TERMINAL OBJECTIVE

To be able to state the indications and contraindications for convulsive therapy and to use the treatment safely in psychiatric disorders.

ENABLING OBJECTIVES

1. *Be able to identify the various types of convulsive and subconvulsive therapies currently used and be able to state and discuss for each:*

① *1.1. Indications and contraindications*

② *1.2. Technique of the procedure*

Guide: Include how to decide on number of treatments.

① *1.3. Precautions and hazards and how these are minimized*

① *1.4. Efficacy*

② *1.5. The modifications of the "classical" bipolar method and the results with modified procedures (e.g., unilateral)*

③ *1.6. Mode of action (theoretical), including biochemical and dynamic theories.*

Guide: Include:

1.6.1. Emphasis on electroconvulsive therapy (ECT)

1.6.2. Others

　　　1.6.2.1. Pharmacoconvulsive (Indoklon)

　　　1.6.2.2. Nonconvulsive electronarcosis

　　　1.6.2.3. . . .

　　　1.6.2.4. . . .

1.7. Interactions with other treatments (dangers and precautions)

      1.8. . . .
      1.9. . . .
   2. . . .
   3. . . .

C. Psychosurgery

TERMINAL OBJECTIVE

To know the indications and to be able to select appropriate patients for lobotomy and other psychosurgical procedures.

ENABLING OBJECTIVES

1. Be able to discuss the current status and methodology of psychosurgery as a "treatment" (attitudes and controversy) and be able to state the:

③   *1.1. Anatomical and physiological mechanisms involved*
③   *1.2. Indications and contraindications*
③▼③▲ *1.3. Criteria for selection of patients*

      Guide: By the psychosurgical conference

③▼③▲ *1.4. Postoperative and aftercare procedures*
③▼③▲ *1.5. Complications*
③   *1.6. Therapeutic results*
③   *1.7. Rationale of the psychosurgical therapy*

      Guide: Types of psychosurgery:
      a. Standard lobotomy
      b. Modified lobotomy
      c. Transorbital lobotomy
      d. Thalamotomy
      e. Cingulectomy
      f. Temporal lobectomy
      g. Stimulation of thalamic centers
      h. Stimulation of other centers
      i. . . .
      j. . . .

   2. . . .
   3. . . .

D. Miscellaneous and Little-Used Biological Treatments

ENABLING OBJECTIVES

1. Be able to state the reported (or reputed) indications in psychiatric practice and the current professional opinion about each of the following types of treatment:

④   *1.1. Subcoma insulin therapy*

④   *1.2. Drug-induced abreactive states*
④   *1.3. Continuous sleep therapy (narcosis)*
④   *1.4. Hormone treatments*
④   *1.5. Vitamin treatments*
④   *1.6. Physiotherapy*
④   *1.7. Hydrotherapy*
    1.8. . . .
    1.9. . . .
2. . . .
3. . . .

Section XV. Learning Theory and Behavior Modification

GENERAL PLAN

A. Learning Theory
B. Behavior Modification

A. Learning Theory

TERMINAL OBJECTIVE

To acquire a working knowledge of learning theory as it applies to the understanding of personality development and psychiatric disorders.

ENABLING OBJECTIVES

③   *1. Be able to state and describe the major tenets of "S–R" theory (behaviorism) and its clinical application, including:*
    1.1. Contributions of major theorists

        Guide:
        1.1.1.   Guthrie, E. R. (theory of learning)
        1.1.2.   Hull, C. L. (habit family hierarchy)
        1.1.3.   Pavlov, I. (classical conditioning)
        1.1.4.   Skinner, B. F. (operant conditioning)
        1.1.5.   Thorndike, E. (law of effect)
        1.1.6.   Tolman, E. C. (theory of learning)
        1.1.7.   Watson, J. B. (conditioned reflex theory)
        1.1.8.   Miller, N. E. (applications of biofeedback)
        1.1.9.   . . .
        1.1.10. . . .
②   *1.2. Classical conditioning*

        Guide:
        1.2.1.   Eysenck, H. J. (personality testing, introversion–extraversion)
        1.2.2.   Pavlov, I. (classical conditioning)
        1.2.3.   Wolpe, J. (clinical application, reciprocal inhibition)

1.2.4. . . .
1.2.5. . . .

③   *1.3. Operant conditioning*

    Guide:
    1.3.1. Skinner, B. F. (operant conditioning)
    1.3.2. . . .
    1.3.3. . . .

③   *1.4. Personality development*

    Guide:
    1.4.1. Bandura and Walters (social learning)
    1.4.2. Dollard and Miller (social learning, functional amnesia)
    1.4.3. Mowrer, O. H. (two-factor learning theory)
    1.4.4. . . .
    1.4.5. . . .

    1.5. Fundamental concepts:
        1.5.1. Stimulus
        1.5.2. Response
        1.5.3. Reinforcement
        1.5.4. Schedules of reinforcement
        1.5.5. Conditioning
        1.5.6. Learning
        1.5.7. Extinction
        1.5.8. Spontaneous recovery
        1.5.9. Discrimination
        1.5.10. Generalization
        1.5.11. "Law of effect"
        1.5.12. . . .
        1.5.13. . . .

③   *1.6. Cognitive theory*
        1.6.1. Development
            1.6.1.1. Piaget, J. (stages of development)
            1.6.1.2. . . .
            1.6.1.3. . . .
        1.6.2. Personality and therapy

        Guide:
        1.6.2.1. Beck, A. (scale for depression)
        1.6.2.2. Ellis, A.
        1.6.2.3. Kelly, G.
        1.6.2.4. Lazarus, A.
        1.6.2.5. . . .
        1.6.2.6. . . .

    1.7. . . .
    1.8. . . .

  2. *Where appropriate for each subject in objective 1 above, be able to discuss the subject under the following headings:*

④   *2.1. Experimental evidence*
③   *2.1.1. In animals*
③   *2.1.2. In humans*
③   *2.2. Application to clinical psychiatry*
③   *2.3. Knowledge of the technical terms appropriate to the theory*

     3. Be able to state some of the recent advances in our understanding of the neurophysiological basis of learning.

     4. Be able to discuss the present state of knowledge concerning:

④   *4.1. The issue of "choice" in human behavioral change*
④   *4.2. The implications of learning theory for social change*
③   *4.3. The implications of learning theory for preventative mental health programs*
③   *4.4. Biofeedback*
            4.5. . . .
            4.6. . . .
     5. . . .
     6. . . .

B. Behavior Modification

TERMINAL OBJECTIVE

To learn the effective and ethical application of the principles of learning in the treatment of psychiatric disorders.

ENABLING OBJECTIVES

     1. For each of the commonly used techniques in the behavioral therapies, be able to state:

③*   *1.1. The method of the procedure*
③*   *1.2. The theoretical rationale and the elements in the procedure*
③†   *1.3. The indications and contraindications for the procedure*
③†   *1.4. The therapeutic outcome studies (results)*
            1.5. . . .
            1.6. . . .

           Guide:
           a. Desensitization (including counterconditioning)
           b. Reciprical inhibition and desensitization
           c. Conditioned avoidance
           d. Aversive conditioning
           e. Extinction
           f. Negative practice (exhaustion)
           g. Flooding

*At a .01 to .1 level of significance each of these has a priority ranking of ▽②△.
†At a .03 and .06 level of significance, respectively, these two objectives have a priority ranking of ▽②△.

        h. Modeling

        i. Behavioral rehearsal (role-playing)

        j. Relaxation therapy

        k. Biofeedback

        l. Assertive training

       m. Token economies

        n. Thought stopping

        o. Multimodel behavior therapy

        p. . . .

        q. . . .

  1.7. . . .

  1.8. . . .

2. *Be able to:*

  2.1. *Assess the patient's problems to determine whether one or more of the behavioral therapies is appropriate and, if it is, to define the goals of therapy and the evaluation criteria.*

  2.2. *Design the procedure. Specify the behaviors to be modified, and the consequences to be applied to those behaviors, and the contingency relationship between the behaviors and consequences. Specify the procedures used to facilitate the contingency relationship.*

  2.3. *Implement the therapy procedures with the patient's knowledge and consent.*

  2.4. *Evaluate the therapy:*

    2.4.1. *In consultation with the supervisor, determine whether the design and procedures have been properly and consistently implemented.*

    2.4.2. *Evaluate the behaviors of interest to determine whether they are changing in a manner consistent with the originally stated goals.*

  2.5. *If stated goals are not being attained, begin the decision process again at step 2.1, and change some aspect (goals, design, procedures) to achieve the identified goal.*

  2.6. . . .

  2.7. . . .

3. *For the technique of biofeedback, be able to state (see also Section X, objective 4.1):*

  3.1. *Objectives 1.1.–1.4. above, stressing the importance of each in the treatment of psychosomatic illnesses*

  3.2. *Research findings relating to voluntary control of functions subsumed under the autonomic nervous system*

  3.3. . . .

  3.4. . . .

4. . . .

5. . . .

Section XVI. The Psychotherapies

GENERAL PLAN

A. Individual Psychotherapy
B. Group Psychotherapy
C. Family Psychotherapy
D. Psychotherapy with Children
E. Milieu Therapy
F. Activity and Rehabilitation "Therapies"

TERMINAL OBJECTIVES

1. To be able to demonstrate a general understanding of the underlying theoretical principles and hypotheses behind each of the major psychotherapeutic techniques.
2. To be acquainted with all major psychotherapeutic techniques including the behavior therapies, understand the advantages and limitations of such techniques, and be capable of drawing from the basic principles underlying any and all of them in the "process" of treatment.
3. To develop an appreciation, through experience, of one's abilities and difficulties in using such techniques.
4. To develop an ability to relate psychotherapeutically to all age levels and diagnostic groups.
5. To appreciate the ethical issues involved in all areas of the practice of psychotherapeutic intervention.

ENABLING OBJECTIVES FOR ALL PSYCHOTHERAPIES

① *1. Be able to demonstrate a psychodynamic understanding of the psychotherapeutic relationship(s), how it is started, formed, terminated, stages therein, and how the relationship may be disrupted.*
① *2. Be able to demonstrate skill in assessment of patients for psychotherapy techniques.*

   Guide: Indications, contraindications.
① *3. Be able both to state and to demonstrate a working knowledge of the underlying principles, assumptions, and hypotheses on which each treatment modality is based by being able to correctly "prescribe" the appropriate treatment(s) and set realistic goals for each.*
① *4. Be able to demonstrate, with clinical material, skill in interpretation, reflection, clarification, support, empathy, and confrontation.*
② *5. Be able to demonstrate, in the clinical setting, an awareness of the effects on the therapeutic process of those biases in both the therapist and the patient that arise from cultural stereotypes of male and female behavior.*

②   *6. Be able to review critically modern studies on the effectiveness of the various types of psychotherapy.*

     Guide: Include being able to make "critical" statements concerning:

     a. Principles and methods of research, including such topics as reproducibility, generalizability, ethics, design, controls, and criterion measures.

     b. Improvement without treatment

     c. Outcome variables:

        Treatment method

        Diagnosis

        Demographic variables (patient)

        Motivation and expectancy (patient)

        Attitude (patient)

        Mental status (patient)

        Qualifications of therapist (including experience) and "school" or orientation

        "Personality" and demographic background of therapist

        Temporal variables

        Personality compatibility of the therapist and patient

        The social, cultural, and physical setting

     d. Results of adequately controlled studies

     e. . . .

     f. . . .

7. . . .

8. . . .

A. Individual Psychotherapy

ENABLING OBJECTIVES APPLICABLE TO TREATMENT MODELS IN GENERAL

1. Perceptual and conceptual skills: Be able to:

     1.1. General

①   *1.1.1. Recognize and describe patient–therapist interaction.*

①   *1.1.2. Give a dynamic description of a patient appropriate to the treatment model.*

①   *1.1.3. Recognize and describe effects of patient on one's self.*

        1.1.4. . . .

        1.1.5. . . .

     1.2. Re the patient

①   *1.2.1. Where appropriate, conceive of symptoms as motivated by conflicts (unconscious and other) that are to be identified.*

①   *1.2.2. Assess the patient's ability to change.*

①   *1.2.3. Recognize and describe resistance.*

①▽□△   *1.2.4. Define key concepts operationally.*

          1.2.5. . . .

          1.2.6. . . .

        1.3. Re the therapist

①▽□△   *1.3.1. Deal with feelings about being a therapist.*

①▽□△   *1.3.2. Become aware of how one's personal characteristics influence how one becomes a therapist.*

②   *1.3.3. Assess the effectiveness of one's approach, particularly interpretations made.*

          1.3.4. . . .

          1.3.5. . . .

        1.4. . . .

        1.5. . . .

      2. Executive skills: Be able to:

①   *2.1. Establish contact and stimulate rapport.*

①   *2.2. Set objectives and contracts with the patient.*

        2.3. Clarify communication by interpreting:

②   *2.3.1. Resistance*

②   *2.3.2. Affect*

②   *2.3.3. Transference*

        2.3.4. . . .

        2.3.5. . . .

②   *2.4. Help the patient label affect, then link affect and insight.*

①   *2.5. Help the patient understand interactions with the therapist.*

①   *2.6. Recognize and deal with countertransference.*

②   *2.7. Develop a* therapy style *consistent with one's personality.*

        2.8. . . .

        2.9. . . .

③   *3. Supervisory skills: Be able to demonstrate skills in supervising junior colleagues by:*

        3.1. Exhibiting an openness to understanding other "styles" without the need to impose any particular model

        3.2. Assisting the junior colleague in analyzing:*

②   *3.2.1. The theme of the hour*

①   *3.2.2. The patient's dynamics, defenses, and behavior*

②▽□△   *3.2.3. Alternative therapeutic interventions—their pros and cons*

②▽□△   *3.2.4. Timing and focus of interpretations*

①▽□△   *3.2.5. Issues of support vs. confrontation*

②   *3.2.6. Issues of detachment vs. involvement*

②   *3.2.7. Degrees of therapist activity*

②▽□△   *3.2.8. Nonverbal communication (by both therapist and patient)*

---

*The prototype manual on goals and objectives on which the priority rating questionnaire for 3.2 was based read: "Have supervision which deals with. . . ." All ratings are for *that* original question. The original manual was not accompanied by a log book. This item was considered "experiential" and therefore moved to the Log Book (Chapter 2), and the objective modified to cover supervisory skills.

①▽☐△   *3.2.9.   The therapist's own conflicts that interefere with his therapeutic efficiency*

         3.2.10. . . .

         3.2.11. . . .

     3.3. . . .

     3.4. . . .

   4. . . .

   5. . . .

ENABLING OBJECTIVES APPLICABLE TO SPECIFIC TREATMENT MODELS

1. For a minimum of the treatment models listed in subobjectives 1.1–1.5 below, be able to define:

①   *a. Selection criteria for appropriate patients*

①   *b. The theoretical principles and hypotheses on which the model is based*

①   *c. The appropriate use of the technique in terms of the objectives for the patient (or the stage in the therapeutic process)*

     Guide: Establishing therapeutic alliance, setting contracts, reducing excessive anxiety, reducing negative behavior, relieving symptoms, establishing reality principles (roles), taking responsibility for self, reclaiming projections, stopping maladaptive repetitive transactional behavior patterns, correcting and reestablishing "internalizations," reestablishing basic trust and practicing adaptive thinking, feeling, and behavior.

①▽☐△   *d. The method of application*

②▽☐△   *e. Principal terms*

     Guide: Note, in particular, the terms listed under subobjectives 1.1–1.5 inclusive.

①▽☐△   *f. The principal limitations of the technique, including contraindications to its use*

①▽☐△   *g. The probable outcome*

     Guide: Include "critical" reference to evaluation studies for at least subobjective 1.2.

     h. . . .

     i. . . .

①*   *1.1. Supportive psychotherapy (long-term and short-term)*

     Guide: Adaptive defenses, suppression, corrective emotional experience, and restoration of a state of "equilibrium"

     1.2. Psychoanalytically oriented psychotherapies

②*   *1.2.1. Brief*

②*   *1.2.2. Focal*

---

*At levels of significance ranging from .06 to .1 the trend continues for the American respondents to give a priority of 2 vs. the Australians' 3 or 4.

③*   *1.2.3. Psychoanalysis*

   Guide: Include knowledge about:
   a. Therapeutic alliance
   b. Transference
   c. Interpretation, clarification, and confrontation
   d. Insight
   e. Countertransference
   f. Working through
   g. Resistance
   h. Acting out (acting in)
   i. The negative therapeutic reaction
   j. Principle of "focusing" (on a topic)
   k. Principle of "minimal activity"
   l. . . .
   m. . . .

④   *1.3. Transactional analysis and structural analysis*

   Guide: Include knowledge about:
   a. Ego state (e.g., parent, adult, child)
   b. Contamination and exclusion
   c. Existential position
   d. Strokes
   e. Transactions (e.g., complementary, crossed, angular, duplex)
   f. Time structuring (games, rackets, stamps)
   g. Script
   h. Contract (goal direction)
   i. . . .
   j. . . .

④   *1.4. Gestalt therapy (Perls, F.)*

   Guide: Include:
   a. Concept of awareness
   b. Experiencing the "gestalt"
   c. Figure and ground separation
   d. . . .
   e. . . .

④   *1.5. Other "psychotherapies"*
   1.5.1. Specialized techniques for the treatment of sexual dysfunctions
   1.5.2. Reality (Glasser)—concept of responsibility
   1.5.3. Primal (Janov)—concept of abreaction
   1.5.4. Client-centered (Rogers)
   1.5.5. Morita therapy
   1.5.6. Bioenergetics, structural reintegration

*At levels of significance ranging from .06 to .1 the trend continues for the American respondents to give a priority of 2 vs. the Australians' 3 or 4.

> 1.5.7. *Massage*
> 1.5.8. *"Centering"—yoga*
> 1.5.9. *Transcendental meditation*
> 1.5.10. *Art therapies*
> 1.5.11. *Occupational therapy*
> 1.5.12. *Rational emotive therapy*
> 1.5.13. . . .
> 1.5.14. . . .
> 1.5.15. . . .
> 1.5.16. . . .
> 1.5.17. . . .

B. Group Psychotherapy

ENABLING OBJECTIVES APPLICABLE TO GROUP TREATMENT APPROACHES IN GENERAL*

② 1. *Be able to demonstrate comfort and competence in dealing with a wide variety of groups, approaches, and techniques.*

② 2. *Be able to list and discuss indications and contraindications for group therapy.*

② 3. *Be able to demonstrate physical and mental ease in relating to patients and colleagues in group situations.*

② 4. *Be able to specify and describe the dynamics exhibited by persons in group situations.*

> *Guide:* Include:
> a. Milieu therapy
> b. Group therapy
> c. Team meetings (colleagues)
> d. Large group meetings (colleagues)

② 5. *Be able to demonstrate an ability to recognize and use therapeutically the nonverbal communications seen in group situations.*

② 6. *Be able to identify and describe approaches appropriate for different categories of groups and the types of patients appropriate for each approach.*

   7. *Be able to demonstrate competence in:*

②   7.1. *Working effectively in staff conferences, ward milieu groups, etc.*
②   7.2. *Working as a member of a team*
②   7.3. *Working in leadership roles in a group*
②   7.4. *Serving in a consultant role to various groups such as social agencies*
        7.5. . . .
        7.6. . . .

   8. . . .
   9. . . .

*All the objectives (1–7) in this section are given a lower priority ranking by the Australian respondents.

ENABLING OBJECTIVES APPLICABLE TO SPECIFIC
GROUP TREATMENT APPROACHES

①   *1. For a minimum of the treatment models listed in subobjectives 1.1–1.7
    below, be able to discuss:*
②   *a. Selection criteria for patients*
③   *b. Composition of groups*
③   *c. Pros and cons for selection of, use, and misuse of a cotherapist (where
       appropriate)*
③   *d. Type of leadership (include discussion re leaderless groups)*
③   *e. Time factors (including "marathon")*
③   *f. Methodology*
③   *g. Theoretical principles and hypotheses on which the model is based*
③   *h. Principal limitations of the technique, including contraindications
       for its use*
③   *i. Probable outcome (including "critical" reference to evaluation studies)*
    j. . . .
    k. . . .
③   *1.1. Group therapy utilizing primarily one or more (any combination) of
         the techniques listed in objective 1 under Topic A, ENABLING
         OBJECTIVES APPLICABLE TO SPECIFIC TREATMENT
         MODELS*
③   *1.2. "Classical" group therapy, i.e., the therapy of the individual within
         the group (analytically oriented psychotherapy, psychodrama, and
         so on) (e.g., Freud, Wolf and Schwartz, Morino)*
③   *1.3. Group therapy by the "interpersonalists," i.e., the study of the inter-
         action among the individuals in the group, transactional analysis,
         and so on (e.g., Eric Berne)*
③   *1.4. Group therapy by the "integrationists," i.e., the study of the group
         and the group process as a whole (e.g., Bion)*
④   *1.5. Combined approaches (e.g., Ezriel, French, Yalom)*
④   *1.6. Specialized groups: Sensitivity or "T," encounter, crisis models*
③   *1.7. Other models*
         1.7.1. Educational model
         1.7.2. Milieu model and therapeutic community
         1.7.3. . . .
         1.7.4. . . .
    2. . . .
    3. . . .

C. Family Psychotherapy*

ENABLING OBJECTIVES

③   *1. Be able to discuss the current theoretical hypotheses and concepts that
    underlie the various types of family therapy and the historical develop-
    ment of these approaches.*

*All objectives (1–4) in this section are given a lower priority ranking by the Australian respon-
 dents (level of significance .007 to .2).

Guide:
a. Ackerman, N. W.
b. Boszormenyi-Nagy, I.
c. Bateson, G.
d. Bowen, M.
e. Epstein, N.
f. Haley, J.
g. Jackson, D.
h. Laing, R.
i. Lidz, T.
j. Satir, V.
k. Wynne, L. C.
l. . . .
m. . . .

② 2. *Be able to identify and evaluate the illness of family member(s) in the context of his/her/their family.*

③ 3. *Be able to do a family assessment and describe a family systematically.*

Guide: Include pertinent statements on the following factors:
a. Diagnostic formulation, including specific psychopathology of each member where appropriate
b. The social, cultural, and physical (e.g., housing) environment of the family and the changes that have occurred in these factors over the past two generations
c. The marital "contract," both covert and overt
d. Autonomy (quality, degree of, reaction to it in other members)
e. Roles (e.g., traditional, idiosyncratic–scapegoat, binder, discharge)
f. Communications (clarity, directness, and qualifiability; affective, instrumental, and information-sharing)
g. Affect identification, experiencing, and handling
h. Problem identification, -solving, and relationship of problem-solving to homeostasis
i. Equilibrium (homeostasis and its relationship to all the foregoing, to patterns of interaction, to shared pathology and defenses, to reinforcing patterns, and so on)
j. The family's ability to respond positively to the therapist's interactions with them
k. Health as a "universal" (rather than a culturally relative) phenomenon
l. . . .
m. . . .

③ 4. *Be able to demonstrate an ability to carry out the psychotherapeutic treatment of families.*

Guide: By means of both treating a number of families in long-term therapy under supervision and demonstrating competence in teaching family therapy by having supervision of one's supervision of junior residents, be able to:

4.1. Utilize all techniques listed in objective 1 under Topic B, EN-ABLING OBJECTIVES APPLICABLE TO SPECIFIC GROUP

TREATMENT APPROACHES, and in objective I under Topic A. ENABLING OBJECTIVES APPLICABLE TO SPECIFIC TREATMENT MODELS, as they appear to be appropriate to the treatment of specific families.

4.2. Recognize and label the effect on one's self of interactions and transactions with the family.

4.3. Demonstrate the relationships between interactions and transactions and the symptoms.

4.4. Engage a family in a therapeutic contract that the family understands and be able to articulate a management plan.

4.5. Help the family work out specific new adaptive patterns capitalizing on strengths and resources.

4.6. Interrupt and alter the system of family functioning.

4.7. Reward new adaptive behaviors as they occur.

4.8. Set tasks and help the family to work on them.

4.9. Work on individual dynamics where necessary.

4.10. Recognize and deal with common shared disturbing affective issues in a family and work them through to some conclusion.

4.11. Demonstrate a range of techniques combined with a knowledge and an awareness of any personal tendencies to overreact and miss affects and be able to use these techniques in a flexible way related to a sensitivity to one's own and the family's internal use.

4.12. Progress from observing nonverbal affective tones of transactions to hypothesizing their function and then entering into the family system to change them.

4.13. Change hunches that do not check out.

4.14. . . .

4.15. . . .

5. . . .

6. . . .

D. Psychotherapy with Children

ENABLING OBJECTIVES

③ 1. *Be able to demonstrate knowledge about and competence in all the objectives in Topics A–C as they apply to the treatment of children and their families.*

② 2. *Be able to discuss the role of developmental processes as they pertain to the treatment of the child.*

Guide: Include:

a. Pathological processes

b. Healthy processes and, as such, innate personal resources of the child, which can be enhanced by the psychotherapeutic process

c. Communication skills, including verbal, nonverbal, level of concep-

tualization attainable, and, most significantly, the role of play as a
major modality of child psychotherapy

　　d. The positive as well as negative resources in the child's environment

②　3. *Be able to recognize and differentiate problems that are primarily intra-
psychic in origin and problems that have their transitory foundations in
extrapsychic situations.*

③　4. *Be able to demonstrate competence in the psychotherapeutic treatment
of the child and his/her family.*

　　Guide: By means of having had a minimum of three long-term experiences throughout the residency program with families, preferably starting
just prior to or after the birth of a child, and with older sibs if possible,
in addition to having a minimum of two supervised experiences doing
play therapy with a child, the postgraduate should be able to demonstrate:

　　4.1. Knowledge of the general meaning of play and its therapeutic usefulness

　　4.2. Skill in forming a therapeutic working alliance with a child

　　4.3. Knowledge of different phases of psychotherapy and their meaning
for children

　　4.4. An ability to set appropriate developmentally relevant goals

　　4.5. Knowledge of the limits of child psychotherapy and of his own limits
in the practice thereof

　　4.6. Skill in working with children in groups

　　4.7. Skill in working with parents, both directly and in collaborative
work with other professionals (including "supportive" psychotherapy, "education" of parents, and so on)

　　Guide: Develop "rapport" and have empathy.

　　4.8. . . .

　　4.9. . . .

5. . . .

6. . . .

E. Milieu Therapy

ENABLING OBJECTIVES

1. *Be able to work efficiently, effectively, and harmoniously both as a member and as a leader of a mental health team in the:*
　　1.1. *Inpatient setting*
　　1.2. *Outpatient setting*
　　　　a. *in information-gathering*
　　　　b. *in treatment-planning*
　　　　c. *in the application of various therapeutic regimens*

2. *Demonstrate, in a clinical setting, an ability to define the milieu in operational terms.*

　　Guide: Include:
　　2.1. Boundaries

2.2. Stages of the group process and its effect on the individual patient
2.3. The milieu as a "system" (see Section IV.E, objective 4.3)
2.4. Therapeutic factors:
    2.4.1. Potential effects thereof
    2.4.2. Timing of various types of staff–patient and group interactions
2.5. Drawbacks and limitations
2.6. Patient selection—indications and contraindications
2.7. Potential negative factors:
    2.7.1. Possible effects thereof
    2.7.2. Measures to counteract
2.8. . . .
2.9. . . .
3. . . .
4. . . .

F. Activity and Rehabilitation "Therapies"

ENABLING OBJECTIVES

1. For the following treatment approaches:
    1.1. Vocational workshop and counseling programs (hospital)
    1.2. Vocational rehabilitation programs (community-based)
    1.3. Occupational therapy programs (hospital)
    1.4. Community "occupational therapy" programs
    1.5. Recreational and physical fitness programs
    1.6. "Educational" programs (other than vocational rehabilitation)
    1.7. "Camping" and outward-bound-type programs
    1.8. "Self-help groups"
    1.9. . . .
    1.10. . . .
be able to operationally define each type of program and describe a typical example. Include:
a. Indications, contraindications, and patient selection
b. Advantages

    Guide: Physical, psychological, and sociological
c. Potential drawbacks

    Guide: Physical, psychological, and sociological
d. Typical or expected outcome and limitations with different "groups" (diagnostic) of patients
e. Cost benefit
f. . . .
g. . . .
2. . . .
3. . . .

Section XVII.   Community and Administrative Psychiatry*

GENERAL PLAN

A. Historical Development and Definition
B. Basic Psychiatric Principles
    i. The Concept of Prevention
    ii. Continuity of Care
    iii. Large-Group Dynamics
    iv. Team Functioning
C. Basic Administrative Principles
    i. Regionalization
    ii. Systems Theory
    iii. Management
    iv. Audits of Patient Care
D. Methods of Intervention
E. Research

TERMINAL OBJECTIVE

To be able to combine what is known concerning the biological, psychological, social, cultural, and environmental factors that affect both individuals and groups with concepts of primary, secondary, and tertiary prevention, to create and maintain an adequate health care delivery system in the community.

A. Historical Development and Definition

ENABLING OBJECTIVES

③   *1. Be able to review, briefly but critically, the historical development of community psychiatry, noting in particular the quodlibet concerning community psychiatry as: "standard treatment practices transported to a different setting" vs. "a new philosophy and concept of care."*
    2. Be able to state the relevance of current social phenomenona to the mental health of the population involved.
        2.1. "Structure," e.g., poverty, living conditions, cultural or minority grouping, employment opportunities
        2.2. Process—movements (e.g., black power, women's lib)
        2.3. . . .
        2.4. . . .

---

*The objectives in this section for the most part are given priority rankings of 3 or 4. The Canadian respondents, however, ranked these objectives 2 or 3, respectively. These differences did not reach a .01 level of significance.

④ *3. Be able to discuss briefly major contributions to community psychiatry.*

    Guide: Include:
    a. Coles, R.
    b. Jones, M.
    c. Kennedy, J. F.
    d. Kaplan, G.
    e. Paumelle, P.
    f. . . .
    g. . . .

4. . . .

5. . . .

B. Basic Psychiatric Principles

i. The Concept of Prevention

ENABLING OBJECTIVES

② *1. Be able to define (with examples) primary, secondary, and tertiary prevention and list modalities commonly used in each type in modern psychiatric practice.*

③ *2. Be able to list and state the primary mandate of the major community human resources in your locality.*

    Guide: A suggested organization of resources is as follows:
    2.1. Health
    2.2. Education
    2.3. Social and community services
    2.4. Justice
    2.5. Corrections
    2.6. Local community human services
    2.7. Other or "unavailable" resource categories

③ *3. Taking into consideration all commonly used demographic population categories (e.g., age group, sex) for each community resource area and for the group of resources as a whole, be able to state the role of their component parts in:*
    3.1. Primary prevention
    3.2. Secondary prevention
    3.3. Tertiary prevention

③ *4. Be able to discuss the importance of a "sense of community" in urban and rural settings.*

    Guide: Note in particular:
    4.1. The homonomous and autonomous drives of individuals and groups
    4.2. Process and effects of isolation, alienation, etc.
    4.3. Fulfillment of fundamental needs of individuals (e.g., Maslow's hierarchy) and of groups

    4.4. Effects of "prosperity" and depression

    4.5. . . .

    4.6. . . .

② 5. *Be able to review critically the effects of "institutionalization."*

    Guide: Dependency, effects of separating sexes, age groups, and so on. For example, Goffman's work.

  6. *Be able to state and discuss factors relating to hospital "readmission" rates.*

    Guide: Community adjustment —the relative importance of "symptoms" vs. the patient's ability to structure time constructively and usefully.

  7. . . .

  8. . . .

ii. Continuity of Care

ENABLING OBJECTIVES

1. *Be able to discuss the principle of continuity of care from the point of view of:*

②   *1.1. The patient*

②   *1.2. The professional*

③   *1.3. The health care administrator*

    Guide: Note where appropriate the effects of such factors as:

    a. Separation from known environment, physical and interpersonal

    b. Multiple therapists, both simultaneous and consecutive, with respect to delineation of responsibility, effectiveness of therapies, efficiency, etc.

    c. "Tracking" mechanisms; their therapeutic and administrative uses

    d. . . .

    e. . . .

2. . . .

3. . . .

iii. Large-Group Dynamics

ENABLING OBJECTIVES

③ 1. *Be able to relate common community or large-group defenses such as dominance, territoriality, and other theme interference defenses to the perpetuation of gaps and duplications in and fragmentations of the human services delivery system in a prescribed area.*

2. . . .

3. . . .

iv. Team Functioning

ENABLING OBJECTIVES

1. Be able to discuss the team approach (both interdisciplinary and multi-agency), including:

③   *1.1. Definition of role (e.g., clearly delineated roles vs. role diffusion, typical roles of each discipline)*

③   *1.2. Definition of responsibility (e.g., accountability, of leaders, of members)*

③   *1.3. Membership change (e.g., realignment of roles)*

③   *1.4. Communication processes*

③   *1.5. Problem-solving mechanisms*

③   *1.6. Affect-handling mechanisms*

③   *1.7. The illusion of "team"*

     1.8. . . .

     1.9. . . .

2. Be able to discuss the advantages and disadvantages of the treatment team working primarily in the community from the point of view of:

③   *2.1. The patient (as an individual, as a group)*

③   *2.2. The professional: clinical and administrative, service, education, and research*

     2.3. The community

     with respect to:

③   *a. Effectiveness, coordination, role diffusion*

③   *b. Efficiency, cost benefit*

     c. . . .

     d. . . .

3. . . .

4. . . .

C. Basic Administrative Principles

i. Regionalization

TERMINAL OBJECTIVE

To be able to discuss the concept of regionalization as it pertains to the delivery of mental health services.

ENABLING OBJECTIVES

③   *1. Be able to discuss the influence of minority groups, cultural or socioeconomic or both, on the design for delivery of services for a given region.*

④   *2. Be able to state and critically discuss resource needs for a given "catchment" area.*

Guide: Include:
a. Persons in each mental health discipline per 100,000 population and for what purposes
b. Mental health facilities of each major type per 100.000 population
c. Beds allotted for both acute and chronic care per 100,000 population

Ⓐ 3. *Be able to discuss the similarities and differences in designing a viable delivery system for mental health services in:*
   3.1. A rural setting
   3.2. An urban setting
   3.3. A rural–urban setting

   Guide: Organization of services, types of services, other resources, manpower, etc.

Ⓐ 4. *Be able to state the viable size of a "region" (total population, population density, geographic area) for a given quantity of resources.*
   5. . . .
   6. . . .

ii. Systems Theory

ENABLING OBJECTIVES

Ⓐ 1. *Be able to apply systems theory in explaining succinctly how changes in one section of the community affect functioning in other sectors where sectors include not only the "human services" sectors listed in Topic B.i, objective 2, above but also the business, political, and other sectors.*

Ⓐ 2. *Be able to describe succinctly deficits in the service delivery system with special reference to primary, secondary, and tertiary prevention in the area, and suggest methods for correcting same without increasing total dollar expenditure within that service system.*

Ⓐ 3. *Be able to outline and discuss factors that tend to decrease the effectiveness of current attempts to coordinate human services.*
   4. . . .
   5. . . .

iii. Management

ENABLING OBJECTIVES

1. *Be able to state the principal tenets of and the pitfalls in:*
Ⓐ   *1.1. Matrix management*
Ⓐ   *1.2. Management by objectives*
      1.3. Other management systems
      and indicate briefly how they can be utilized in the design and maintenance of a comprehensive system for:
Ⓐ   *a. The delivery of clinical services in a mental health complex (multidisciplinary)*

④   b. *The delivery of human services in a community of 50,000 or more*
             population (multiagency, multidisciplinary)

2. . . .

3. . . .

iv. Audits of Patient Care

ENABLING OBJECTIVES

④   1. *Be able to design an objective and comprehensive method for auditing*
          patient care.

      Guide:
      a. The medical or clinical record
      b. The quality of treatment of individual cases
      c. The effectiveness of the service delivery system

2. . . .

3. . . .

D. Methods of Intervention

ENABLING OBJECTIVES

③   1. *Be able to discuss methods of intervention particularly relevant to the*
          practice of community psychiatry.

      Guide: Include:
      1.1. Family therapy (cf. Section XVI.C)
      1.2. Small-group therapy (cf. Section XVI.B)
      1.3. Large-group intervention relating to such activities as:
          1.3.1. Mobilization and integration of resources (e.g., N. Hansell)
          1.3.2. Decodification of client–group communications (e.g., R.
              Speck)
          1.3.3. Ecosystem approaches for ameliorating external sources of
              tension (e.g., M. Morekv)
          1.3.4. Task-oriented or work groups (e.g., W. Bion; cf. Section
              XVI.B, ENABLING OBJECTIVES APPLICABLE TO
              GROUP TREATMENT APPROACHES IN GENERAL,
              objective 1.4)
      1.4. Crisis intervention (cf. Section IX.A)
      1.5. . . .
      1.6. . . .

③   2. *Be able to define, describe, and demonstrate competence in at least four*
          distinct types of consultation (e.g., Caplan's).

      3. *For each of the following alternative treatment settings or any combina-*
         tion thereof:
         3.1.   *Outpatient (clinic)*

3.2. *Day or evening care (center)*
3.3. *Home care*
3.4. *Group home*
3.5. *Foster home*
3.6. *Camp (or camping), farm*
3.7. *Halfway house*
3.8. *Inpatient*
    3.8.1. *Children's treatment center*
    3.8.2. *Hospital or equivalent*
    3.8.3. *Nursing home or equivalent*
3.9. *. . .*
3.10. *. . .*
be able to describe a typical example and state:
a. *Indications (factors governing selection of patients)*
b. *Contraindications*
c. *"Dangers" (including factors concerning length of stay, position in social system and family, community attitudes, and employment)*
d. *Typical outcome (discuss limitations)*
e. *Factors that influence readmission*
f. *. . .*
g. *. . .*

4. *Be able to compare and contrast the settings listed in objective 3 above.*
   Guide:
   a. Efficacy for defined problems
   b. Limitations
   c. Necessary personnel
   d. Cost
5. *. . .*
6. *. . .*

E. Research

ENABLING OBJECTIVES

1. *Be able to outline the methods of investigation and the principal conclusions of epidemiological and sociological research pertinent to community practice of psychiatry, including:*

③   1.1. *Research relevant to the prevalence of mental illness (e.g., Midtown Manhattan Study, Stirling County Study)*

    1.2. *Research relevant to the relationship between:*

③   1.2.1. *Prevalence of mental illness and social class (e.g., Hollingshead and Redlich)*

③   1.2.2. *Prevalence of mental illness and degree of social integration (e.g., Stirling County Study, A. Leighton)*

③▽②⚠   1.2.3. *Mental illness and migration*

        1.2.4. *. . .*

        1.2.5. *. . .*

1.3. . . .
1.4. . . .
2. . . .
3. . . .

Section XVIII.   Geriatric and Forensic Psychiatry

GENERAL PLAN

A. Geriatric Psychiatry
B. Forensic Psychiatry
    i. Psychiatry and Criminal Law
    ii. The Concept of Competency
    iii. Compulsory Detention and Treatment, Where Applicable, of the
    Mentally Ill

A. Geriatric Psychiatry

TERMINAL OBJECTIVE

    To learn how to evaluate, diagnose, and treat psychiatric illnesses occurring in the geriatric age group.

ENABLING OBJECTIVES

①   *1. Be able to describe the process of aging, its stages and crises, as part of developmental psychology and sociology (e.g., retirement).*
①   *2. Be able to do a competent assessment of a geriatric patient, including:*
       2.1. A general assessment of the "physical" status and a detailed psychiatric assessment
       2.2. History, which should include special attention to present life circumstances (such as physical illness, recent losses, and supportive elements operating in family and community); mental status, which should emphasize the affective and cognitive changes occurring in the elderly
       2.3. . . .
       2.4. . . .
①   *3. Be able to list and describe common physical and mental disease states of the elderly from the epidemiological, pathological, and clinical points of view.*
①   *4. Demonstrate, in the clinical setting, an ability to relate the specialized usage of psychotropic medications in the elderly, with special attention to indications and contraindications.*
     5. For each of the treatment modalities commonly used in psychogeriatric practice, be able, using clinical examples, to state:
①   *5.1. Realistic objectives*

①   *5.2. Indications*
①   *5.3. Contraindications*
①   *5.4. Side effects*
①   *5.5. Method of application*
       5.6. . . .
       5.7. . . .
       6. *Be able to list and apply specialized techniques for facilitating the geri-*
          atric patient's orientation.

          Guide:
          a. Consistent, predictable environment
          b. Clear delineation of time, of rooms, of dates, of events, etc.
①   7. *Be able to list and discuss the stages of mourning.*
       8. *Using one's theoretical knowledge concerning the process of mourning,*
          demonstrate an ability to manage issues concerning death and dying
          in the clinical setting with respect to:
②   *8.1. The patient*
②   *8.2 The family*
②   *8.3. Other caretakers (e.g., ward nurses)*
②   *8.4. Self*
②   9. *Be able to discuss the reactions of the therapist that prevent function-*
          ing effectively with the elderly.
       10. *. . .*
       11. *. . .*

B. Forensic Psychiatry*

i. Psychiatry and Criminal Law

TERMINAL OBJECTIVE

    To be cognizant of the relationship between criminal law and mental
disorder (illness or retardation).

ENABLING OBJECTIVES

③   1. *By observing a senior psychiatrist acting as expert witness in cases that*
          the resident has had an opportunity to interview or see interviewed, be-
          come familiar with court procedures and the current role of a psychia-
          trist in the adversary system.
       2. *Be able to state current state or provincial practices and legislative re-*
          quirements concerning confidentiality and the legal "infringements"
          thereupon.
       3. *Be able to state the legal requirements for:*
②   *3.1. Fitness to stand trial*

*At a level of significance ranging from .02 to .2 Canadians consistently give higher priority to
objectives in this topic area than do Americans or Australians.

②   *3.2. Trial procedures in which the accused is found fit to stand trial but in which there may be evidence of mental illness or retardation and/or personality disorders*

    3.3. . . .

    3.4. . . .

②   *4. Be able to state in detail current tests of criminal responsibility or their equivalent and their application.*

    Guide:

    4.1. McNaughton rule

    4.2. American Law Institute

    4.3. . . .

    4.4. . . .

④   *5. Be able to compare and contrast national rules affecting psychiatric evidence (e.g., American, British, Canadian, Australian).*

    Guide: Include, for example. the McNaughton rule and the Durham rules.

③   *6. Using actual case examples, be able to write a succinct, factual report containing a clearly stated opinion that would be acceptable for court proceedings.*

    7. Be able to state and discuss the procedure(s) by which persons:

③   *7.1. For whom the court requires psychiatric assessment*

③   *7.2. Who are found not fit to stand trial*

③   *7.3. Who are found not guilty by reason of insanity*

    7.4. . . .

    7.5. . . .

    can be placed under psychiatric observation or care or both.

②   *8. Be able to state and discuss the review procedures available for persons held involuntarily in psychiatric facilities.*

    9. . . .

    10. . . .

ii. The Concept of Competency

TERMINAL OBJECTIVE

To examine the concept of competency in relationship to mental illness or retardation.

ENABLING OBJECTIVES

    1. From the standpoint of mental capacity and in the role of expert psychiatric consultant, be able to assess competency in relationship to:

②   *1.1. Contractual capacity*

②   *1.2. Testamentary capacity*

③   *1.3. The marriage contract*

③   *1.4. Tort liability*

③   *1.5. Management of estate*
②   *1.6. Informed consent to submit to medical procedures*
      1.7. . . .
      1.8. . . .
  2. . . .
  3. . . .

iii. Compulsory Detention and Treatment, Where Applicable, of the Mentally Ill

TERMINAL OBJECTIVE

To be familiar with the legislation governing the detention of the mentally disordered.

ENABLING OBJECTIVES

③   1. *Be able to discuss briefly local, national, and international aspects of compulsory detention of the mentally ill.*
         Guide:
         1.1. Statutes
         1.2. For examination, observation, with treatment, without treatment
②   2. *Be able to demonstrate a detailed knowledge of the act(s) or statute(s) applicable within the province of state in which you are practicing that govern:*
         2.1. Rights to treatment
         2.2. Informed consent
         2.3. Competency
         2.4. Review
         2.5. Transfer
         2.6. Child custody
         2.7. . . .
         2.8. . . .
③   3. *See Subtopic B.i, objectives 7 and 8, above.*
      4. *Be able to list and discuss the advantages and disadvantages of applying the principal tenets of the adversary (vs. nonadversary) approach to the compulsory:*
         4.1. Detention of the mentally ill
         4.2. Treatment of the mentally ill
         4.3. Removal of other rights, e.g., to manage own estate
         4.4. . . .
         4.5. . . .
      5. *With respect to the concept of dangerousness, be able to:*
         5.1. Assess it in the clinical setting.
         5.2. State the limits of reliability and validity and the factors bearing thereupon for the clinical assessment of dangerousness.

Section XIX.   Gender and Psychiatry*

Introduction

New work is giving rise to a reframing of the psychology of men and women and to questioning of aspects of theories and treatment models that rest on traditional assumptions about male and female roles. Understanding of these emerging issues is of vital importance to the postgraduate. At present, this section contains more material on women and women's issues, since there is a notable lack in this area related to a prior focus on male development and acceptance of this focus as the norm. It is envisaged that a growing amount of new work will be done on male psychology.

This section also contains far more names of current authors, though only as guides, than any other section.† Again, the inclusion of authors' names was a contentious issue, and the number included here reflects the newness of this area as a focal point for study.

GENERAL PLAN

A. Emerging Issues in the Psychology of Women and Men
B. Sociocultural Aspects
C. Special Issues
D. Psychotherapy

TERMINAL OBJECTIVES

1. To attain a working knowledge of the emerging body of literature on gender identity and gender role which have implications for psychiatric theory and clinical practice.
2. To be cognizant of the effect of sex role stereotypes on theory, practice, and research.

A. Emerging Issues in the Psychology of Women and Men

ENABLING OBJECTIVES

③   *1. Be able to describe the traditional gender role stereotypes, i.e., those personality traits, characteristic behaviors, and characteristic psychopath-*

*The priorities for this section were obtained by a separate questionnaire. No comparison between nations has been carried out on these data.
†The reference list is included in Appendix D.

*ologies that have been commonly believed to be more characteristic of
the one sex or the other in the twentieth-century Western world.*

Guide: Consider:
a. Broverman (clinical stereotyping)
b. Gore (sex roles and mental illness)
c. . . .
d. . . .

2. *Be able to state for each "role" noted in objective 1 above whether it is
   disconfirmed, or remains unclear in the present state of knowledge, with
   respect to the following behaviors:*

③ 2.1. *Aggression*
③ 2.2. *Nurturant behavior*
④ 2.3. *Mathematical and verbal abilities*
③ 2.4. *Achievement behavior and motivation*
③ 2.5. *Sexual drive and behaviors*
③ 2.6. *Depression*
③ 2.7. *Alcoholism and abuse of prescription drugs*
③ 2.8. *Sociopathy*
③ 2.9. *"Hysteria" and hypochondriasis*
   2.10. . . .
   2.11. . . .

3. *Be able to define and contrast gender identity and gender role behavior,
   including:*

② 3.1. *Critical developmental stages*
② 3.2. *The ages at which these stages typically occur*
   3.3. . . .
   3.4. . . .

Guide: Consider:
a. Money and Ehrhardt (biological basis of gender identity)
b. Stoller (sex and gender)
c. . . .
d. . . .

4. *Be able to summarize current knowledge of the determinants of:*

② 4.1. *Gender identity*
② 4.2. *Gender role behavior*
   4.3. . . .
   4.4. . . .

5. *State major contributions of recent authors to the understanding of male
   and female life cycles and the similar and different stresses typical of
   each.*

③ 5.1. *Prenatal*

Guide: Parental preferences

③ 5.2. *Infancy and toddlerhood*

Guide: Attachment; bonding, core gender identity

③ 5.3. *Preschool*

Guide: Early recognition of gender role

③ 5.4. *Early school years*

Guide: Sex separation in peer group play

③ 5.5. *Preadolescence*

Guide: Biopsychology of cyclic changes, divergence of cognitive styles between boys and girls, psychosexual development, hetero-sexual awareness

③ 5.6. *Later adolescence*

Guide: Adaptation and consolidation, subcultures, career choice

③ 5.7. *Early adulthood*

Guide: Vocation, marriage, child-rearing, fears of gynecological pathology, goal conflicts, therapeutic termination of pregnancy

③ 5.8. *Middle adulthood*

Guide: "Second career," recognition of the body "deterioration," "last-chance-to-succeed" feeling, divorce, adoption, child custody

③ 5.9. *Late "middle age"*

Guide: Menopause, role changes, widowhood, cultural denial of older women's sexuality

③ 5.10. *Old age*

Guide: Loss of health, retirement, death of loved ones (males), financial strains

Guide: Consider the work of such authors as:
a. Baker, Miller (psychology of women)
b. Maas and Kupyers (longitudinal study 30–70)
c. Pleck (male psychology, masculinity)
d. Seiden (research on psychology of women)
e. Tooley (pitfalls of traditional male role)
f. . . .
g. . . .

③ 6. *On the basis of the data above or recent critiques or both, be able to eval-uate critically at least three major theories of personality development and family and group interaction.*

Guide: Consider:
6.1. Freud, S. (theories of psychosexual development)
6.2. Erikson (psychosocial theory)
6.3. Learning theory
6.4. Sullivan (interpersonal theory)
6.5. Maslow (self-actualization)
6.6. Ackerman (family dynamics)
6.7. Theories derived from ethology
6.8. . .
6.9. . . .

7. *Be able to discuss the role of vocational aspirations and work roles and experiences with respect to:*

③   7.1. *Solidifying identity in adolescence, adult life, and the retirement years*

③   7.2. *Discussing possible differences in these issues for males and females*

④   7.3. *Summarizing current data on sex differentials in employment rates, wage scales, advancement opportunities*

③   7.4. *Assessing and managing a problem presented by a woman patient who had been subjected to gender-based discrimination in a work situation*

7.5. . . .

7.6. . . .

Guide: Consider such work as:
a. Commissions on women's status and equality in the United States and Canada
b. Howe (women's traditional occupational world)
c. . . .
d. . . .

8. . . .

9. . . .

B. Sociocultural Aspects

ENABLING OBJECTIVES

④   1. *Be able to discuss and evaluate the history of psychiatry and medicine in relationship to a history of attitudes toward the sexes with regard to work, marriage, family, and psychiatric treatment.*

Guide: Consider:
a. All references for the history of psychiatry
b. History of childhood (Aries and DeMause)
c. Women in historical perspective (de Beauvoir, Mill)
d. History of male and female sex roles in America (Filene)
e. History of fear of women (Hays, *Malleus Maleficarum*)
f. History of women as patients and healers (Ehrenreich)
g. . . .
h. . . .

④   2. *Be able to describe gender roles and related childrearing practices in at least three other cultures.*

Guide: Consider:
a. Bronfenbrenner (families in Russia)
b. Mead (women in primitive societies)
c. Sidel (women and child care in China)

    d. . . .

    e. . . .

④   3. *Be able to state how gender role expectations differ in at least three ethnic subcultures found in the Western world.*

    Guide: Consider the work of such authors as:

    a. Bernard (sociology of the family)

    b. Huber (women in changing society)

    c. . . .

    d. . . .

④   4. *Using clinical case examples or recent research, or both, be able to describe the effects of social context and expectancies on behavior, attitudes, and "labeling."*

    Guide: Utilize knowledge gained from your understanding of the work of some of the following authors:

    a. Goffman (incarceration, labeling of deviant behavior)

    b. Milgram (influence of authoritarian experimenter)

    c. Rosenhan (normal subjects in mental hospital)

    d. Rosenthal (teacher expectation and pupil performance)

    e. . . .

    f. . . .

  5. *With respect to the effect of maternal employment on children, be able to:*

③   *5.1. Summarize current knowledge.*

③   *5.2. Compare this with current knowledge concerning the effects on children of:*

        5.2.1. Paternal employment patterns

        5.2.2. Parental unemployment

        5.2.3. Job changes

        5.2.4. Marital disruption and realignment

        5.2.5. Other life events

④   *5.3. Use your knowledge of child development as well as recent empirical work to contrast effects of factors in subobjectives 5.1 and 5.2 above on children of varying ages.*

④   *5.4. State age-appropriate methods of modifying influences of factors in subobjectives 5.1 and 5.2 above where the evidence suggests they are deleterious.*

        Guide: Consider the work of:

        a. Howell (families of employed mothers)

        b. Eisenberg (parenting dilemmas)

        c. . . .

        d. . . .

    5.5. . . .

    5.6. . . .

  6. . . .

  7. . . .

C. Special Issues*

ENABLING OBJECTIVES

1. *Be able to describe and critically assess the interaction of biological, psychological, social, cultural, and environmental factors in the following areas (use recent contributions to our understanding of male and female psychosexual development and the sociocultural context within which behavior is or is not defined as deviant):*

③   *1.1. Aggression and violence against women*
            Consider:
            1.1.1. Rape and society

                Guide: Brownmiller
            1.1.2. The rape victim

                Guide: Hilberman
            1.1.3. The rapist

                Guide: Cleaver
            1.1.4. Battered wives

                Guide: Martin. Hilberman
            1.1.5. Battered children (with special reference to female adolescents)

                Guide: Gil. Van Stolk
            1.1.6. Generalized violence against women

                Guide: Russell
            1.1.7. Issues in victimology (pitfalls and genuine issues in "blaming the victim"), incest . . .
            1.1.8. . . .
            1.1.9. . . .
③   *1.2. Aggression and violence by women*

            Consider:
            1.2.1. Inhibition of aggression in women

                Guide: Bernardez-Bonnesati, Lerner
            1.2.2. The woman offender

                Guide: Adler, F.
            1.2.3. Battery of children by women
            1.2.4. The woman murderer
            1.2.5. Male and female fears of women's aggression

                Guide: Hays. Lerner
            1.2.6. The issue of "passive aggression"
            1.2.7. Women as alleged or real accomplices or nonprotesting bystanders in cases of aggression by men (with special reference to child abuse, rape, incest)

*Note that these issues are not entirely limited to women, e.g., V.D., circumcision.

           1.2.8. . . .

           1.2.9. . . .

②   *1.3. Sexuality*

        Consider:

           1.3.1. Masturbation (frequency, fantasies, importance in sexual therapy)

             Guide: Kinsey, Dodson. Hite. Kline-Graber)

           1.3.2. Coital function and dysfunction

             Guide: Masters and Johnson. Kaplan. Kline-Graber

           1.3.3. Lesbianism

             Guide: Martin

           1.3.4. Sexuality in later life

             Guide: Busse and Pfeiffer. Kuhn

           1.3.5. Sexual experience in childhood

             Guide: Katchadourian and Hunde

           1.3.6. Sexuality in adolescence

           1.3.7. Effects of psychiatric illness and psychotropic medication on sexuality

           1.3.8. . . .

           1.3.9. . . .

③   *1.4. The menstrual cycle*

        Consider:

             Guide: Dan *et al.*

           1.4.1. Menarche

             Guide: Whisnant

           1.4.2. Menopause

             Guide: Bart

           1.4.3. Premenstrual syndromes

             Guide: Parlee

           1.4.4. Diagnosis and treatment of paramenstrual distress

           1.4.5. Evidence for and against affective, cognitive, perceptual, libidinal, and behavioral changes with the cycle

           1.4.6. Evidence for cyclic biochemical/physiological changes that may alter response to psychotropic medications

           1.4.7. . . .

           1.4.8. . . .

③   *1.5. Fertility*

        Consider:

           1.5.1. Psychology of infertility

           1.5.2. Psychology of family planning

           1.5.3. Contraception (including medical and psychiatric hazards and benefits of various approaches)

　　　　1.5.4. *Abortion (psychological, gynecological, and psychiatric hazards and benefits; relationship to use of other fertility control approaches)*

　　　　　　　Guide: Freeman

　　　　1.5.5. *Sterilization: psychiatric consequences in male and female; indications for and against in psychiatric illness and mental retardation; issues of ethics and informed consent*

　　　　1.5.6. *Fertility and fertility control in adolescents*

　　　　1.5.7. . . .

　　　　1.5.8. . . .

③　1.6. *Pregnancy, childbirth, and lactation*
　　　Consider:

　　　　1.6.1. *Medicalization of childbirth*

　　　　　　　Guide: Arms, Shaw

　　　　1.6.2. *Parent–child bonding*

　　　　　　　Guide: Klaus and Kennell, Brazelton

　　　　1.6.3. *Effects on infant of not being breast fed*

　　　　1.6.4. *Effects of psychotropic medication on fetus and lactating infants*

　　　　　　　Guide: Shader, Smith

　　　　1.6.5. *Effects of obstetric medication on infant, on mother–child bond, and on the initiation of lactation*

　　　　　　　Guide: Brazelton

　　　　1.6.6. *Psychotropic medications (re pseudocyesis, galactorrhea)*

　　　　1.6.7. *Postpartum psychiatric syndromes: incidence; treatment; indications for and against simultaneous hospitalization of mother and child*

　　　　1.6.8. *Pregnancy in adolescence and middle age: obstetric and psychiatric hazards and advantages; incidence of fetal problems*

　　　　1.6.9. *Issues involved in psychiatric consultation re continuation or interruption of pregnancy*

　　　　1.6.10. . . .

　　　　1.6.11. . . .

③　1.7. *Diseases and surgery of the reproductive system*
　　　Consider:

　　　　1.7.1. *Infectious (venereal) diseases in male and female; psychiatric and neuropsychiatric consequences*

　　　　　　　Guide:
　　　　　　　a. Tests for
　　　　　　　b. Management of
　　　　　　　c. Phobias of
　　　　　　　d. . . .
　　　　　　　e. . . .

　　　　1.7.2. *Genetic and developmental defects*

　　　　　　　Guide: Turner's syndrome

   1.7.3. Malignant diseases of reproductive organs:
    1.7.3.1. Psychological consequences of
    1.7.3.2. Hormonal consequences of
    1.7.3.3. Fear of castration in male and female
    1.7.3.4. . . .
    1.7.3.5. . . .
   1.7.4. Psychiatric aspects of surgery on the reproductive organs,
    e.g., hysterectomy, circumcision
   1.7.5. . . .
   1.7.5. . . .
  1.8. . . .
  1.9. . . .
 2. . . .
 3. . . .

D. Psychotherapy

ENABLING OBJECTIVES

③   *1. Be able to state, using clinical case examples or knowledge of research, the effects of clinician bias related to cultural gender role stereotypes on therapeutic process and outcome.*

  Guide: Consider the work of:
  a. Broverman (clinician stereotyping)
  b. Chesler (psychiatry oppressing women)
  c. Smith and David (women's experiences of therapy)
  d. Bonesatti and Lerner (aggression expressed by women in therapy)
  e. . . .
  f. . . .

③   *2. Be able to summarize present knowledge about the effect of a therapist's gender on the process and outcome of psychotherapy.*

  Guide: Consider the work of:
  a. Howard and Orlinsky (recommendations for women patients)
  b. Luborsky (therapist–patient similarity produces favorable outcome)
  c. . . .
  d. . . .

③   *3. Be able to summarize present knowledge about possible adverse effects of psychotherapy with particuliar reference to the relevance of this work to women.*

  Guide: Consider the work of such authors as:
  a. Bergen (evaluation of therapeutic outcomes)
  b. Halleck (politics of therapy)
  c. Strupp (surveys of patients and therapists)
  d. Tennov (hazards of psychotherapy for women)
  e. . . .
  f. . . .

③ 4. *Be able to outline the distinctions between psychiatric illness proper and common situational problems of women more appropriately treated by any or a combination of job counseling, assertiveness training, women's groups, marital counseling, and psychotherapy for the husband.*

     Guide: Consider the work of such authors as:
     a. Franks and Burtle (women in psychotherapy)
     b. . . .
     c. . . .

    5. *Be able to outline a plan for (a) diagnostic assessment and (b) treatment of sexual dissatisfaction or dysfunction in:*
②   *5.1. Patients of both genders*
②   *5.2. Patients of various marital statuses*
②   *5.3. Patients with different object orientations*
     5.4. . . .
     5.5. . . .

     Guide: Consider the work of:
     a. Masters and Johnson (studies of sexual performance)
     b. Kaplan (therapy of sexual dysfunction)
     c. . . .
     d. . . .

    6. *Be able to state ways of recognizing and managing erotic transference and countertransference in psychotherapy, including:*
②   *6.1. Differentiation of erotic, oral-dependent, hostile-dependent transferences, defense transferences, and defenses against transferred feelings*
②   *6.2. Management of patient's transference without narcissistic injury to patient*
②   *6.3. Recognition of therapist's countertransference feelings evoked by patient's transference*
②   *6.4. Recognition of time in therapist's own life cycle when vulnerability to countertransference acting-out is heightened*
②   *6.5. Appropriate preventive and, if necessary, corrective action to be taken for sexual abuse of the therapeutic relationship*
     6.6. . . .
     6.7. . . .
    7. *. . .*
    8. *. . .*

Section XX. Psychiatric Research and Evaluation

GENERAL PLAN

A. History and Philosophy of Psychiatric Research Design
   1. Social and historical factors that influence the definition, diagnosis, and treatment of deviant, illegal, and illness behavior

2. The historical relationship between the economic, legal, and educational aspects of society and psychiatry
3. Relationship of the development of the psychiatric data base, theoretical models, and the research design to changing historical contents of social philosophy, psychological thinking, scientific methodology, and cultural and technical development

B. Models, Statistics, and Computers in Psychiatry
  1. Theoretical models of explanation and prediction
  2. Legitimate use of statistics in research and evaluation
  3. Uses and limitations of computers in simulation experiments, record-keeping, evaluation, and research

C. Psychiatric Epidemiology as Human Ecology
  1. Language of epidemiology
  2. Problems and limitations of epidemiology
  3. The definition of a psychiatric data base with epidemiological value
  4. Relationships of theoretical models to epidemiology
  5. Relationship of psychiatric problems to community context
  6. Relationship of community problems to ecological context

D. Evaluation of Psychiatric Treatment, Treatment Programs, and Training
  1. Research design, data, and interpretation
  2. Relationships of training to evaluation

A. History and Philosophy of Psychiatric Research Design

TERMINAL OBJECTIVE

To develop a continuously questioning behavior.

Note: This terminal objective, which is outlined under GENERAL PLAN above for the sake of completeness, is considered as essential core.

B. Models, Statistics, and Computers in Psychiatry

ENABLING OBJECTIVES

③ *1. Be able to discuss the strengths, weaknesses, compatibility, and incompatibility of the major models of mental health and illness.*

Guide:
1.1. Medical
1.2. Moral
1.3. Psychoanalytical
1.4. Family interactional
1.5. Social
1.6. Sickness
1.7. Antipsychiatry
1.8. . . .
1.9. . . .

③   2. *Be able to classify functional relationships according to the following categories: necessary, sufficient, and contributory causes; predisposing, precipitating, and perpetuating causes.*

    3. *Be able to define and distinguish among:*

③   *3.1. Independent and dependent variables*
③   *3.2. Constructs and variables*
③   *3.3. Causal and correlational relationships*
③   *3.4. Observations and experiments*
③   *3.5. Data and inferences*
③   *3.6. Quantitative and qualitative evaluation of data*
      3.7. Categorical and quantitative data
      3.8. Reliability and validity
      3.9. Different types of validity
      3.10. . . .
      3.11. . . .

③   4. *Be able to define and describe, where applicable, terms commonly used in statistics and research design.*

      Guide:

      4.1.   Scientific method
      4.2.   Operational definition
      4.3.   Random sampling (discuss pragmatic difficulties involved)
      4.4.   Central tendency (and measurements thereof)
      4.5.   Law of parsimony
      4.6.   Statistical significance (describe tests)
      4.7.   Factor analysis
      4.8.   Computer simulation (uses of)
      4.9.   . . .
      4.10.   . . .

    5. *Be able to:*

③   *5.1. Detect insufficient, biased, and noncompatible samples.*
③   *5.2. Recognize the limits of generalization with respect to sampling methodology and theory.*
③   *5.3. Analyze critically the use of descriptive, correlational, and inferential statistics.*
③   *5.4. Compute the following from raw data: mean, median, mode, and standard deviation.*
③   *5.5. Detect misuses of test of statistical significance.*
      5.6. State for each data-summarizing technique listed in 5.6.1–5.6.6 below:
        a. The underlying principles involved in its computation
        b. The appropriateness of its use for specific examples in the literature
        5.6.1. Mean, median, mode
        5.6.2. Standard deviation
        5.6.3. Correlation coefficients
        5.6.4. Analysis of variance

    5.6.5. t-test
    5.6.6. Chi-square
    5.6.7. . . .
    5.6.8. . . .
  5.7. . . .
  5.8. . . .

④   6. *Be able to discuss the use of computers in, and the contributions of computer technology to, psychiatry.*

    Guide:
    6.1. Research evaluation and statistical analysis
    6.2. Record-keeping
    6.3. The audit of clinical records
    6.4. Epidemiological research
    6.5. Bibliographic information and retrieval systems
    6.6. . . .
    6.7. . .

  7. . . .
  8. . . .

C. Psychiatric Epidemiology as Human Ecology

ENABLING OBJECTIVES

③   1. *Be able to define, using examples from psychiatry, the terms commonly used in epidemiological studies.*

    Guide:
    1.1. Incidence rates
    1.2. Prevalence rates
    1.3. Inception rates
    1.4. Expectancy rates
    1.5. Cumulative prevalence rates
    1.6. Mortality rates
    1.7. Standardized measures
    1.8. Case fatality rates
    1.9. Proportionate mortality rate
    1.10. Descriptive epidemiology—hypothesis formation, null hypothesis
    1.11. Analytical epidemiology—hypothesis testing—observational, experimental
    1.12. Retrospective study (case history), advantages and disadvantages of each
    1.13. Prospective study (cohort)
    1.14. Comparability
    1.15. Bias
    1.16. Indices of mental health
    1.17. . . .
    1.18. . . .

③   2. *Be able to describe the uses of epidemiology in psychiatry.*

      Guide: Concerning the elucidation of, for example:
      2.1. Causation of disease
      2.2. Clinical picture and natural history of disease
      2.3. Estimation of individual risk and recovery
      2.4. Planning and measurement of health services for preventive treatment and control
      2.5. . . .
      2.6. . . .

③   3. *Be able to describe briefly the various epidemiological data collection methods and their limitations.*

③   4. *Be able to describe briefly the factors that commonly distort prevalence data.*

③   5. *Be able to describe and discuss the significance of some of the classic psychiatric epidemiological studies.*

      Guide: Include studies by:
      a. Durkheim, E.
      b. Hallgren, B., and Sjögren, T.
      c. Hollingshead, A. B., and Redlich, F. C.
      d. Kallman, F.
      e. Leighton, A. H.
      f. Rennie, T.
      g. Sainsbury, P.
      h. . . .
      i. . . .

    6. *Be able to:*

④   6.1. *Calculate, from raw epidemiological data: prevalence, incidence, expectancy rate.*

④   6.2. *Apply the language and theory of epidemiology to new psychiatric problems.*

③   6.3. *Detect the limitations of official statistics used in the definition of mental illness.*

④   6.4. *Record and interpret a psychiatric data base to facilitate epidemiological studies in one's own clinical practice.*

④   6.5. *Record the data base necessary to distinguish deviance from disease in the individual case.*

④   6.6. *Describe the effects of different models of psychiatric disorders on the epidemiological data used in incidence and prevalence.*

③   6.7. *Differentiate individual, familial, social, and ecological factors in illness.*

      6.8. . . .
      6.9. . . .
    7. . . .
    8. . . .

D. Evaluation of Psychiatric Treatment, Treatment Programs, and Training

ENABLING OBJECTIVES

④ *1. Be able to analyze critically the use of psychometric instruments in evaluation studies.*

Guide:
1.1. Be able to list and discuss psychological tests and social indicators useful in evaluative studies.
1.2. Be able to evaluate a given test in terms of reliability, validity, and standardization.
1.3. Be able to discuss the limits of generalization.
1.4. Be able to discuss the problem of possible misinterpretation of the results of psychometric tests.
1.5. . . .
1.6. . . .

④ *2. Be able to design and conduct, with supervision, a research project.*

Guide: Be able to design a project and collect and interpret data to:
2.1. Evaluate a given aspect (outcome) of one's own clinical work, one's team's, or one's agency's.
2.2. Analyze the effects of clinical, institutional, and ecological factors on the diagnosis. treatment, and prognosis of individual cases.
2.3. Evaluate the effectiveness of a new psychotropic medication.
2.4. . . .
2.5. . . .

④ *3. Be able to discuss the ecological factors and social processes that critically influence mental health policies in general and the definition, organization, maintenance, and evaluation of psychiatric resources in particular.*

Guide:
3.1. Be able to develop and critically analyze evaluation proposals and studies in light of the ecological factors and social pressures that define resources and policies.
3.2. Be able to evaluate research studies from an ethical point of view.
3.3. Be able to evaluate the appropriateness of generalizing a given evaluation study to a specific population (include statistical vs. practical experience).
3.4. . . .
3.5. . . .

③ *4. Be able to analyze critically a research or evaluation paper in terms of:*

Guide:
4.1. Overall design

4.2. Data

4.3. Methodology

4.4. Conclusion

4.5. Inferential logic relating variables to constructs and in drawing conclusions

4.6. Appropriateness of controls

4.7. Generalizability of results

4.8. . . .

4.9. . . .

5. *Be able to critically assess proposed and completed evaluation studies in terms of types of questions they can answer.*

   Guide:

   5.1. Distinguish appropriately among different types of evaluation procedures.

   5.2. Discuss studies in terms of the audiences to whom they will be useful.

   5.3. Analyze studies in terms of the degree to which they reduce uncertainty among alternatives.

   5.4. . . .

   5.5. . . .

6. *Be able to demonstrate an understanding of the interdependence among target populations, activities, and outcomes as operationalized components of evaluations.*

   6.1. *Implications of different subject selection and assignment procedures*

   6.2. *Comparison of different treatment conditions (activities) with emphasis on operationalization and feasibility*

   6.3. *Different outcome measures*

   6.4. . . .

   6.5. . . .

③ 7. *Be able to evaluate critically and realistically one's own process of education and training.*

④ 8. *Be able to list, describe, and discuss various types of evaluation (operations) research.*

   Guide: Include principles, objectives, methodology, and limitations of the major types of operations research:

   a. Structure

   b. Process

   c. Outcome

   d. Cost benefit

9. . . .

10. . . .

ACKNOWLEDGMENTS

The editor expresses sincere appreciation to the following directors of psychiatric residency training programs who have contributed countless hours to the production of the terminal and enabling objectives and without whom this work would not have come to fruition:

Dr. Arthur Amyot
Department of Psychiatry
University of Montreal

Dr. Roger Bland
Department of Psychiatry
University of Alberta
(Previous to 1975:
  Dr. R. R. Runions)

Dr. J. Divic
Department of Psychiatry
University of Ottawa
(Previous to 1975:
  Dr. K. Mills)

Dr. Michael Entwisle
Department of Psychiatry
University of Calgary

Dr. Patrick Flynn
Department of Psychiatry
Dalhousie University

Dr. Robert C. Hicks
Department of Psychiatry
University of Toronto

Dr. Robert Krell
Department of Psychiatry
University of British Columbia

Dr. C. Lamarre
Department of Psychiatry
Sherbrooke University
(Dr. G. Pinard, 1976 . . .)

Dr. Peter Matthews
Department of Psychiatry
University of Saskatchewan

Dr. C. S. Mellor
Department of Psychiatry
Memorial University

Dr. G. Molnar
Department of Psychiatry
McMaster University

Dr. Georges Painchaud
Department of Psychiatry
Laval University

Dr. W. Powles
Department of Psychiatry
Queen's University
(Dr. P. Hoaken, 1976 . . .)

Dr. Raymond Prince
Department of Psychiatry
McGill University

Dr. Quentin Rae-Grant
Department of Psychiatry
University of Toronto

Dr. Tim Yates
Department of Psychiatry
University of Manitoba
(Previous to 1975:
  Dr. H. Prosen)

Appreciation is also expressed to:

Dr. K. Csapo
Department of Psychology
London Psychiatric Hospital

Dr. Ian Hector
Department of Psychiatry
University of Toronto

Dr. Anne M. Seiden   Dr. P. Sue Stephenson
5544 South Woodlawn Avenue   717 West 10th Avenue
Chicago, Illinois 60637   Vancouver, British Columbia

Mary Ellen Walker
Department of Psychology
London Psychiatric Hospital

Special thanks are due to:

Dr. Charles Bowden
Chairman, Committee on Core Curriculum
American Association of Directors of Psychiatric Residency Training

who was the driving force behind the placing of priorities on the objectives, and to the more than fifty psychiatrists in Australia, Canada, Great Britain, and the United States who were specially requested to set a priority on each objective and who put aside the many hours that were necessary to carry out this laborious task.

Chapter 2

Recommended Training Experiences and Skills: A Log Book

Editor's Introduction

Psychiatric education has a broad eclectic base encompassing biological, psychological, social, cultural, and environmental factors. This variety distinguishes psychiatric training from training for other human services professions. This feature, however, also makes it difficult for the novitiate to monitor clearly the kinds of experiences he or she should be having during the training period. A log book in psychiatric education provides one good solution to this problem, and also helps to prevent the natural tendency to skew "choices" for experience according to one's special interests or conscious or unconscious bias. It further offers an indication of the main work in which a skilled psychiatrist should be competent and a satisfying opportunity to demonstrate good clinical practice. The log book is an outline for the purpose of self-logging residency training experiences and accessing the comprehensiveness of those experiences. It is meant to cover a basic minimum of experiences that a resident should have during training. It is not exhaustive, nor does it attempt to outline minimum experiences for subspecialty areas. It would be expected, therefore, that most of the items listed will be checked off within the first half to three quarters of "generalist" training, with more concentration on special areas of interest being attained in the final portions of training.

Using a log book is essentially a matter of checking off experiences and thereby monitoring the comprehensiveness of your training. The log book itself consists of a list of diagnostic entities, specific treatments, special investigations, and other work experiences that the resident should be involved with during basic "generalist" training in psychiatry. What follows here, therefore, is a list of experiences that you should aim to cover in your training experience. Sample recommended numbers of cases have been included. It should be understood

131

that these are suggestions only and must be modified by your supervisors according to your personal needs and the availability of case material.

Some residents will wish in addition to maintain a folder or binder into which case histories may be placed as a more extensive record of specific experiences. One might also include one or two key reprints or literature references bearing on the diagnostic or treatment problem posed by the entity in question. By being extremely critical and placing only the best of one's work and reading in this binder, one will have, on completion of training, a fast, easily referenced, self-meaningful collection of data that can be of great value in preparing for specialty examinations.

Section I. History, Examination, Formulation, and Diagnosis

It is recommended that the resident make a sincere attempt to do at least one *very thorough* "work-up" (including data collection, formulation, differential diagnosis, and management plan) and "follow-up" on each of the syndromes listed here. The major objectives to be met in working up these case histories are to be found in Chapter 1. References to specific objectives in Chapter 1 that apply to this section of the log book are given at the end of this chapter.

In each of the categories listed below, the resident should follow the patient's course for a minimum of 6 months and preferably 1 year and have the opportunity to reassess the patient at least briefly at the end of that time.* To be included, a case summary should also have been reviewed in detail by the supervisor. As with other chapters, the lists and numbers are suggestions only; the training director should add, delete, or modify. The list stands only as a "guide." It is suggested that you make sufficient identification (case number) to be able to subsequently review the chart or your case history. A reminder, however, that the physician must protect the patient's anonymity; thus, names *must not* be used, and identifying facts should be deleted or disguised.

A. Normal

Follow, for a period of 2–3 years, a normal family with one or more children and in which the mother is within her last 3 months of pregnancy at the time of initial assessment. (The family may be followed for less time if one has raised or is raising children, and this experience may be omitted if it was included in previous medical student experience.)

B. Psychiatric Emergencies†

(The recommended number of cases for assessment is in parentheses at the left of each diagnosis.)

---

*Does not apply to conditions listed under Topic B, Psychiatric Emergencies.

†Since the conditions listed under psychiatric emergencies overlap with those in the next topic, Clinical Syndromes, only a brief work-up is expected (sufficient to make a correct diagnosis and initiate treatment).

Category	Identification Code	Completed	Year	Supervisor	Seen in depth but not in direct care of resident
1. General					
(2) Attempted suicide	1. _____				
	2. _____				
(1) Potentially suicidal	_____				
(1) Violent	_____				
(1) Potentially violent	_____				
(1) Acute anxiety (panic)	_____				
(1) Dissociative state	_____				
(1) Psychosocial "disintegration"	_____				
(2) Alcohol intoxication	1. _____				
	2. _____				
(3) Drug "toxicity" (two different types) (includes overdose and delerium tremens)	1. _____				
	2. _____				
	3. _____				
(1) Abstinence syndrome	_____				
2. "Functional" Psychoses (Acute Emergency)					
(1) Acute paranoid state	_____				
(2) Acute affective state Manic	1. _____				
	2. _____				
Depressed (severe but not necessarily psychotic)	1. _____				
	2. _____				
(2) Acute schizophrenic state	1. _____				
	2. _____				
3. Organic Confusional States					
(1) Delirium (other than due to street drugs)	_____				

Category	Identification Code	Completed	Year	Supervisor	Seen in depth but not in direct care of resident
(1) Epileptic (psychomotor)	_____				
(postictal)	_____				
(1) Hallucinosis (other than drug-induced)	_____				
(1) Amnestic syndrome	_____				

C. Clinical Syndromes (other than in emergency situations)

i. Adult and Adolescent

1. Liaison psychiatry (Supervision should include "style" of presentation to other medical specialists.)

Category	Identification Code	Completed	Year	Supervisor	Seen in depth but not in direct care of resident
(1) Conversion "hysteria"	_____				
(2) Other disorders without demonstrable organic findings but that suggest physical illness	1. _____ 2. _____				
(4) Physical conditions in which psychological factors are considered to be of major importance in the initiation, continuation, or exacerbation of the symptoms (four different organ systems)	1. _____ 2. _____ 3. _____ 4. _____				
(1) Postoperative psychosis	_____				
(1) Postpartum psychosis	_____				

2. Anxiety and Depression

Category	Identification Code	Completed	Year	Supervisor	Seen in depth but not in direct care of resident
(1) A "specific" phobia	_____				
(1) A "generalized" phobia (agora or social)	_____				
(2) Obsessive–compulsive "neurosis"	1. _____ 2. _____				

Category	Identification Code	Completed	Year	Supervisor	Seen in depth but not in direct care of resident
(2) Anxiety of "pathological" degree	1. _____				
	2. _____				
(4) Depression (nonpsychotic)* (four of various degrees of severity)	1. _____				
	2. _____				
	3. _____				
	4. _____				
3. Personality Disorders Including Drug and Psychosexual					
(4) Personality disorders (different diagnostic subtypes including antisocial)	1. _____				
	2. _____				
	3. _____				
	4. _____				
(1) Disorder of "impulse" control	_____				
(1) Chronic "alcoholic"	_____				
(1) Chronic drug-use disorder	_____				
(2) Psychosexual disorders (different diagnostic subtypes)	1. _____				
	2. _____				
4. The "Functional" Psychoses					
(2) Paranoid disorders† (different diagnostic subtypes)	1. _____				
	2. _____				
(6) Schizophrenic disorders (four of different diagnostic subtypes)	1. _____				
	2. _____				
	3. _____				

*The focus of the log book is on *breadth* of experience. A resident will, for example, see many more depressions than the four that he checks off here and enters into his personal case book.

†Classified here for convenience and in keeping with the organization of other parts of this guide.

Category	Identification Code	Completed	Year	Supervisor	Seen in depth but not in direct care of resident
	4. _____				
	5. _____				
	6. _____				
(3) Affective disorders (psychotic) Manic	_____				
Depressed	_____				
"Bipolar" (circular)	_____				
(1) "Reactive/ psychogenic/ borderline psychosis"*	_____				
5. Organic Disorders (Include detailed supervised neuro- logical examinations in four cases.)					
(2) Dementia (middle age and elderly)	1. _____				
	2. _____				
(1) Tardive dyskinesia	_____				
(1) Korsakoff's psychosis (if possible)	_____				
(2) Other organic brain syn- dromes of different etiologies	1. _____				
	2. _____				
(2) Mental retardation[†,‡] Child	_____				
Adult	_____				

*Classified here for convenience and in keeping with the organization of other parts of this guide.
†In these cases, it is suggested that a final follow-up interview be done in 3–6 months after the initial assessment if no further change is expected in the patient's condition.
‡To include etiological factors other than organic.

Category	Identification Code	Completed	Year	Supervisor	Seen in depth but not in direct care of resident

ii. Adolescent

(4) (three different diagnostic categories)
1. _____
2. _____
3. _____
4. _____

iii. Child

1. Pervasive Developmental Disorders
   (1) Autistic child _____
   (1) Childhood "schizophrenia" _____
   (1) Attention-deficit disorder with hyperactivity _____

2. Specific Developmental Disorders
   (2) Learning disorders (different subtypes)
   1. _____
   2. _____
   (1) Other (such as enuresis, encopresis) _____

3. Conduct Disorders
   (1) Undersocialized (including antisocial) _____
   (1) Aggressive _____
   (1) "Nonaggressive" (including runaway) _____
   (1) Socialized (delinquent subculture) _____
   (1) Oppositional (including passive–aggressive and passive–dependent)

Category	Identification Code	Completed	Year	Supervisor	Seen in depth but not in direct care of resident
4. Anxiety Disorders					
(1) School phobia	_____				
(1) Other (e.g., separation anxiety, shyness, withdrawing)	_____				
5. Other (optional) Examples: Stereotyped movement disorder (e.g., Gilles de la Tourette)	_____				
Speech disorders	1. _____				
	2. _____				
	3. _____				
D. Other					
1. (1) Assessment(s) for court	_____				
2. Eating Disorders (adult and/or child) (1) Anorexia nervosa	_____				
(1) Obesity	_____				

Notes:

1. On completion of Section I above (case histories), one will have completed approximately 90 assessments. Somewhat more than half these assessments will include follow-up data from a reassessment interview carried out 6 months or more after the initial assessment.
2. By completing Section I, the resident will have accomplished most, if not all, of Sections II, III, and IV.
3. In order that Sections II, III, and IV not become an *additional* horrendous task, it is suggested that when each case history is completed, a cross-check with Section II, Treatment, Section III, Special Investigations, and Section IV, "Special" Experiences, be carried out to check off appropriate items. In this way, as one reaches the third or fourth year of training, experiential deficiencies will become blatantly obvious.

Section II. Treatments

The resident should have several hours of individual supervision each week in addition to other forms of supervision (e.g., group, case conference). Again, type, time, and place of such supervision are totally within the jurisdiction of the program director and supervisor, and no general statement applies to all centers.

Treatment Modality Type	Dose	Index to Case File	Date Rx Initiated	Date Rx Terminated

A. Organic Therapies

  i. Psychopharmacology

    1. Major Tranquilizers (five chemically different)

Phenothiazines (any two types)				
Butyrophenone				

    2. Metallic Salts (two cases including work-up)

Lithium				

    3. Anxiolytics (two chemically different)

    4. Antidepressants
      Tricyclics and tetracyclics (three chemically different)
      (10 cases minimum)

Treatment Modality Type	Dose	Index to Case File	Date Rx Initiated	Date Rx Terminated
5. MAOI (one case)				
6. Stimulants Methylphenidate (for attention-deficit disorders with hyperactivity) (Optional)				
7. Anti-Parkinsonian Agents (two chemically different)				
8. Sedative/Hypnotics (optional)				
9. Other Disulfiram (one) Methadone (or equivalent) (optional)				
10. Combination Therapy (two cases) (specify which agent used and doses)				

ii. Electroconvulsive Therapy

(including work-up and the obtaining of a written consent) (where available) (12 cases)

Bilateral				
Unilateral				

Treatment Modality Type	Dose	Index to Case File	Date Rx Initiated	Date Rx Terminated

iii. Sodium Amytal Interview

(including the obtaining of a written consent) (one case)

iv. Other and Optional*

Examples:
Electrosleep

Psychosurgery (case work-up or follow-up)

B. Psychotherapies

In this section, to list all the variables such as age, social class, and sex, in addition to all the different types and subtypes of therapy—dynamic, behavioral, experiential, and so on—would have resulted in an impossibly complex grid. Nevertheless, the resident should attempt to obtain a breadth of experience in early training. To this end, it is suggested that the type and the subtype of therapy, for example:

Type	*Subtype*
Dynamic	Classical psychoanalysis, etc.
Behavioral	Reciprocal inhibition, rational therapy, etc.
Experiential	Existential, gestalt, etc.

in addition to the diagnosis and a few basic demographic variables such as age, sex, social class, and ethnic origin be logged for each case. The resident should also attempt to have supervised psychotherapeutic experiences with male and female patients from the upper, middle, and lower social classes, and from the following broad age groupings: 0–20, 20–40, 40–60, and over 60. Accomplishing the foregoing will assure that the resident has carried out all the basic general types of therapy with patients who differ widely in diagnosis, age, and social class.

*See Chapter 1, Section XIV.D, objective 1.

It is also recommended that for each of the following psychotherapy experiences, the resident attempt to have a proportion (e.g., one in eight) of the sessions, including the initial assessment, viewed by a supervisor (live or by video, or both).

Index to Case File	Diagnosis	Type or Subtype	Therapy	Age	Sex	Social Class	Ethnic Origin	Date Therapy Initiated	Date Therapy Terminated	Total Number of Sessions

i. Individual*

  1. Long-term (greater than 18 months, once or more per week) psychodynamically oriented (two cases with different diagnoses; also suggested and in addition: one psychotic and one "borderline")

  2. Long-term (less than above) "supportive" (four cases)

   Psychotic patient (two cases) (18 months or more)

   (two cases with different diagnoses, one being neurotic)

  3. Short-term psychodynamically oriented (two cases with different diagnoses)

*Two cases should be followed to termination.

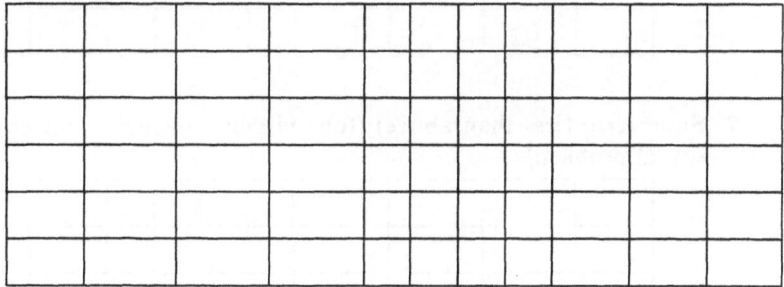

Index to Case File	Diagnosis	Type or Subtype	Therapy	Age	Sex	Social Class	Ethnic Origin	Date Therapy Initiated	Date Therapy Terminated	Total Number of Sessions

4. Short-term "focal" with a specific circumscribed goal (two cases with different diagnoses)

5. Crisis intervention (six cases)

6. Other (two cases using "models" of psychotherapy different from those referred to above, two with adolescent, and one with a latency age child; total five cases) (see Section XVI.A, ENABLING OBJECTIVES APPLICABLE TO SPECIFIC TREATMENT MODELS, objectives 1.3–1.5)

ii. Child—"Play Therapy" (one case)

Index to Case File	Diagnosis	Type or Subtype	Therapy	Age	Sex	Social Class	Ethnic Origin	Date Therapy Initiated	Date Therapy Terminated	Total Number of Sessions

iii. Family Therapy*

  1. Long-term (greater than 1 year) with at least weekly sessions for a reasonable period of time (two families and two couples)

  2. Short-term (less than above) (four families, including one couple with a sexual problem)

  3. Crisis intervention (four cases)

*Two cases followed to termination.

	Comments	Date	Index to Personal Case File
iv. Group Therapy (as Therapist and Cotherapist)			

For the following group therapy experiences, the resident should state the types of techniques he is using, e.g., T.A., Gestalt, and the objective thereof (see Section XVI.A, ENABLING OBJECTIVES APPLICABLE TO SPECIFIC TREATMENT MODELS, objectives 1.1–1.5).

1. Supportive, open (i.e., membership changes with time) (one group, once a week for 6 months or more)

Optional (additional groups)

2. Supportive, closed (membership constant for "life" of group) (minimum one group, once a week, for 6 months or more)

3. Time-limited group (one)

4. Long-term (more than 6 months) psychodynamically oriented "closed" group (one)

5. Other (open or closed using other modalities of treatment, e.g., transactional, educational, role playing, psychodrama)
   Specify type:

6. Other and optional
   Personal experience as group member

Balint type group training

		Index to Personal
Comments	Date	Case File

C. Milieu Therapy

1. A 6-month (or greater) experience as a member and an integral part of a multidisciplinary team on an "in-patient" unit, where at team meetings (preferably weekly) the effects of the "milieu" on the progress of the patient *and* the group of patients is considered in a "defined" manner (one experience)

2. Optional (additional experience)

D. Activity and Rehabilitation Therapies

Plan a treatment program and carry out an evaluation of its outcome with an occupational therapist and a recreational and/or a vocational "therapist" for two patients.

1.			
2.			

Index to Case File	Diagnosis	Type or Subtype	Therapy	Age	Sex	Social Class	Ethnic Origin	Date Therapy Initiated	Date Therapy Terminated	Total Number of Sessions

E. Behavior Therapies

1. With a qualified therapist, carry out four different behavior therapy techniques.
   Desensitization (one patient)

   Biofeedback (one patient)

   Operant conditioning program

Index to Case File	Diagnosis	Type or Subtype	Therapy	Age	Sex	Social Class	Ethnic Origin	Date Therapy Initiated	Date Therapy Terminated	Total Number of Sessions

Optional

2. Follow and "evaluate" the progress of one patient in a "token economy" program.

F. Other and Optional Therapies

1. Hypnotherapy

2. | | | | | | | | |
3. | | | | | | | | |

		Index to Personal
Comments	Date	Case File

Section III. Special Investigations

A. Diagnostic Procedures*

A visit to each laboratory and supervised experience in interpretation of data therefrom:

1. Hematology

2. Biochemistry

3. Skull X rays

4. Computerized axial tomographic scans

5. CSF

*Reference: Chapter 1, Section XIII, objective 5.

	Comments	Date	Index to Personal Case File
6. Urinalysis			
7. EEG			
8. _____			
9. _____			
10. _____			

B. Psychological Tests

Under the supervision of a psychologist, participate in the administration and scoring of six psychological tests; include at least one each of an intelligence test, a personality test, and a test for organicity.

1. _____			
2. _____			
3. _____			
4. _____			
5. _____			

C. Psychophysiology Laboratory Measures
(where available)

Follow four patients through testing procedures involving psychophysiological response patterns.

1. Galvanic skin response			
2. Measures of muscle tension			
3. _____			
4. _____			

Section IV. "Special" Experiences*

A. Home Visits

Six home visits, preferably to homes of patients both of a different social class and of a different cultural background from that of the resident. Five of

*Reference: Chapter 1, Section XVII, Community and Administrative Psychiatry.

		Index to Personal
Comments	Date	Case File

these visits should be carried out and documented in detail in conjunction with an experienced professional of another discipline, such as:

1. A social worker			
2. A public health nurse			
3. A member of the police department			
4. A community occupational therapist (optional)			
5. A child care worker			
6. _____			

B. Experience with Other Human Services Disciplines

In addition to the home visit section above, the resident should assess cases or run a group as a cotherapist with members of other disciplines, such as:

1. A social worker			
2. A psychiatric nurse			
3. A psychologist .			
4. An occupational therapist			
5. _____			

C. Experience with Other Human Services "Agencies" or Centers

1. A working knowledge of the functioning of other human services agencies. Visit on more than one occasion, preferably organized around a mutual client, six of the following:

1.1. City police			
1.2. Probation			
1.3. Juvenile and family court			
1.4. Group home			
1.5. Nursing home			
1.6. Halfway house			
1.7. Youth center (drop-in)			

	Comments	Date	Index to Personal Case File
1.8. Child and family service agency			
1.9. Special education class			
1.10. Overnight hostel for indigents			
1.11. Residential treatment center for children			
1.12. Prison or jail			
1.13. Sheltered workshop			
1.14. Alcoholics Anonymous meeting			
1.15. _____			
1.16. _____			

2. For one or more of the centers listed above, also have a supervised experience in offering a mental health consultation service, concerning:

   2.1. The organization of that agency for effective, efficient service delivery

   2.2. The organization of the human services delivery system as a whole

   2.3. Staff "problems" within that agency

D. Supervision of Junior Colleagues and Other Mental Health Care Workers

   1. Ongoing supervision of junior residents over a period of 6 months

   2. Supervision of other mental health care workers

	Comments	Date	Index to Personal Case File

It is assumed that the resident will have a minimum of 6 months' experience working in:

	Comments	Date	Index to Personal Case File
A general hospital psychiatric unit			
A general hospital outpatient unit			
A children's psychiatric unit Or an equivalent "combined" rotation			

Where available, a resident should also endeavor to have an experience in:

A mental hospital (e.g., state or provincial)			
Or equivalent experiences in an alternate setting			
And 3 months on a neurological service or supervision by a neurologist in another setting			

Where the experiences above are not available, the resident should carefully assess with his training director how equivalent experience can be obtained.

E. Research Experience

Participation in clinical data collection and/or extraction or evaluation of data from records and/or work-up and reporting of clinical cases for publication and/or administration of special clinical interview scales or rating procedures and/or involvement in planning for a research project and/or other (specify)

1. _____			
2. _____			

F. Involvement in a Journal Club for Two or More Years

1. _____			
2. _____			

Suggested Cross-References to Chapter 1

For Section I. History, Examination, Formulation, and Diagnosis

Section	Title	Objective Number	Essence of Objective
II	Normality and Normal Psychosexual Development		
A		2, 3	Assessment of normality
VII	Theories of Personality and Psychopathology		
A		4	Writing a case history
B		4	Concept of "self"
C		3	Use of learning theory
		4	Effects of stress
		5	Repetitive behavior patterns
		7*	Formulation of cases*
VIII	Psychiatric Assessment		
A		8	Empathy and rapport
		9	Information-gathering
		10	Techniques
B		1*	The psychiatric examination*
		3	Formulation using lab test results
		4	Assessment of a family (See also Section XVI.C)
		6	Presentation of data
IX	Psychiatric Emergencies and Reactive Disorders		
A		1	Assessment
B		1	Types of emergencies
C		6, 9	Estimation of suicide potential
D.i		1	Adjustment to stress
D.ii		1	Assessment of grief
		2	Planning management of pathological grief

*Represents a "key" objective.

Section	Title	Objective Number	Essence of Objective
X	Psyche and Soma and Liaison Psychiatry		
		3*	Assessment of patients in whom psychological factors play a major role in the onset or continuation of their physical symptoms*
		4.2	Education of patients
		4.4	Setting of objectives for "intervention"
XI	The Neuroses, Personality Disorders, Addictions, and Sexual Disorders		
GENERAL . . .		2	Assessment and formulation
SPECIFIC . . .			
A		1	Dynamic formulation of a case (See also Section VII.C, obj. 7.)
B		3	Goal-setting
C		5, 7	Diagnosis and treatment of alcoholism
D		1	"Formulation" of sexual deviations
XII	The "Functional" Psychoses		
. . . ALL PSYCHOSES: CLINICAL		1	Interview and assessment and planning of management
F		4	Differential diagnosis, mental retardation and clouding of consciousness
XIII	The Organic Mental Disorders		
		5, 6	Assessment (including laboratory investigations)

*Represents a "key" objective.

Section	Title	Objective Number	Essence of Objective
XVI	The Psychotherapies		
. . . ALL PSYCHO-THERAPIES		1–5	Interview and assessment
C		3	Assessment of a family
XVIII	Geriatric and Forensic Psychiatry		
A		2	Assessment of a geriatric patient
B.i		3, 6	Psychiatric assessment (including fitness) for a report to the court
B.ii		1	Assessment of competency

For Section II. Treatments

Section	Title	Objective Number	Essence of Objective
VI	Child and Adolescent Psychiatry		
A.i		2	Therapeutic approaches child and family
A.iv		5	Therapeutic approaches to the adolescent
A.v		2	Family therapy
B		4	Therapy and team approach
C		5–8	Genetic counseling
IX	Psychiatric Emergencies and Reactive Disorders		
C		9	Treatment of a potentially suicidal patient
D.i		3	Types of management (brief)
D.ii		2	Management of pathological grief
X	Psyche and Soma and Liaison Psychiatry	3.5	Treatment of psychosocial complications
		4	Treatment of psychological factors in physical illness

Section	Title	Objective Number	Essence of Objective
XI	The Neuroses, Personality Disorders, Addictions, and Sexual Disorders		
SPECIFIC . . .			
A		3	Therapeutic approaches
B		2	Therapeutic approaches
C		5	Treatment of abstinence syndrome
		7	Therapeutic approaches
D		2	Therapeutic approaches
XII	The "Functional" Psychoses		
. . . ALL PSYCHOSES: GENERAL		5	Therapeutic approaches
		6	Team approach
		7	Prognostic indicators
		8	Prevention
XIII	The Organic Mental Disorders		
		6	Planning of treatment
XIV	The Organic Therapies*	All*	
XV	Learning Theory and Behavior Modification		
A		2.2	Application
B		1	Techniques
		3.1	Biofeedback
XVI	The Psychotherapies*	All*	Includes individual, group, family, children, milieu, and activity and rehabilitation*
XVII	Community and Administrative Psychiatry		
B, C		All	Service delivery systems
D		All	Consultation

*These objectives are of major importance.

Section	Title	Objective Number	Essence of Objective
XVIII	Geriatric and Forensic Psychiatry		
A		4	Psychotropic medication
		5	Treatment approaches
		6	Technique for facilitating orientation
		8	Management of the dying patient

Because all the following sections overlap and interrelate, the specific objectives have not been listed or repeated after each of the conditions listed in the log book section.

Section	Title

For Section III. Special Investigations

VIII	Psychiatric Assessment
XIII	The Organic Mental Disorders

For Section IV. "Special" Experiences

XVII	Community and Administrative Psychiatry

ACKNOWLEDGMENTS

Grateful acknowledgment is made for the encouragement and guidance given by Dr. G. F. Heseltine, Professor and Chairman, Department of Psychiatry, University of Western Ontario, London, Ontario, Canada, and to Dr. Harold Merskey, Professor and Director of Education and Research, London Psychiatric Hospital, for his critical review of early drafts.

Chapter 3

The Residency Training Program Audit

Editor's Introduction

One of your prime concerns as a resident is what your particular training center can offer you in terms of breadth of generalist training, depth of training available in your chosen specialty area, and the quality of each. Residents should be involved both individually and as a group in evaluating and monitoring these aspects of their training program. Four areas may be considered: (1) the structure of the program (a measure of quantifiable items such as core subject areas, resources, and supervised experiences); (2) the process (a judgment of the manner in which the available physical resources, clinical material, and the expertise of the staff are being utilized by the postgraduates); (3) the outcome of the program; and (4) the cost benefit. The latter two evaluatory processes, i.e., outcome and cost-benefit analysis, will not be considered in detail here.

The following questions represent one means for carrying out a relatively comprehensive program audit. If they are used in the form of a survey of a particular program, then it is useful to compare opinions of residents and staff. Although for quantitative purposes specific criteria can be set for each question listed herein, the editor's preference is to leave the questions open-ended. In this form, many of the questions here may be used as a guide by potential residents when they are attempting to assess different residency training programs with a view to making an application for training.

This audit outline is one suggested method for making a program review, and again, specific questions asked will have to be modified by the residents in conjunction with their training director according to the specifics of their own programs.

Section I. General

1. Does the program meet national standards for an approved psychiatric residency training?

    Yes_____ No_____

2. How many residents are in each year of the program?

    1st: _____ 2nd: _____ 3rd: _____ 4th: _____

Section II. Structure

	Yes	Somewhat	No	Comments
1. Can a physician observer clearly understand the relationship between the objectives of the program and the learning experiences to which the resident is exposed?				
2. Can a physician observer clearly understand the method by which the following are carried out?				
2.1. Evaluation of residents				
a. Knowledge				
b. Skill				
c. Attitudes				
2.2. Evaluation of the program				
a. Structure				
b. Process				
c. Outcome (optional)				
d. Cost benefit (optional)				
3. Have objectives for learning been clearly outlined in areas of knowledge, skill, and attitude?				
4. Is the resident told on entering the program roughly where, when, and how he will receive experience in each of the major areas outlined in the objectives for training (e.g., acute care, long-term care, child and adolescent psychiatry, geriatric psychiatry)?				
5. Are there adequate facilities for training— for example:				
5.1. Office space?				
5.2. Secretarial services?				
5.3. Equipment (e.g., audiovisual aids)?				
6. Is there a clear method for selection of trainees?				
7. Is there a clear method for selection of staff?				
8. Is there a clear method for evaluation of staff:				
8.1. By peers?				
8.2. By residents?				

	9A			Comments	9B		
	Yes	Somewhat	No		Yes	Somewhat	No

9. Does the resident (A) have access to and (B) make adequate use of (a "process" question):

9.1. A library with a sufficient selection of texts and journals and with a capability to access other major medical libraries and "search" services such as Medlars?

9.2. Staff, supervisors, clinical chief of service, education committee and each of its members, and the departmental chairman?

9.3. Training experiences in both inpatient and outpatient settings?

9.4. Training experiences with other specialties, such as:
  a. Neurology?
  b. Emergency medicine?
  c. Family practice?
  d. Social work?
  e. Psychology?
  f. Clinical psychophysiology?
  g. Other?

9.5. Training experiences in subspecialty fields, such as:
  a. Child psychiatry?
  b. Adolescent psychiatry?
  c. Geriatric psychiatry?
  d. Family and group dynamics and therapies?
  e. Psychiatric emergencies and crisis intervention?
  f. Psychosomatic medicine and liaison psychiatry?
  g. Special types of theory and therapy—for example:
    g.1. Psychodynamic psychotherapies?
    g.2. Behavioral therapies?
    g.3. Experiential therapies?

	9A				9B	
Yes	Somewhat	No	Comments	Yes	Somewhat	No

h. Community psychiatry?
i. Administrative psychiatry?
j. Forensic psychiatry?
k. Research (basic)?
l. Research (operative)?
m. Other

	Yes	Somewhat	No	Comments

10. How many hours of supervision per week do residents receive:

Individually? _____

In group? _____

11. Is there a log book or some other such objective mechanism for outlining required experiences during residency training?

12. Is there at least an annual review with each resident and the director of training or the chairman or both to ascertain the postgraduate's progress as per the log book (see Chapter 2) and the supervisor's reports and to receive feedback from the residents concerning the adequacy of the program?

Section III. Process

1. A. Do the residents know what is expected of them—for example, by means of:
   A.1. Objectives?
   A.2. Log book?
   A.3. Personal communication?
   B. Are the residents given adequate feedback—for example, by means of:
   B.1. Regular supervisor's verbal reports (minimum every 3 months)?
   B.2. Regular supervisor's written reports (minimum every 6 months)?
       and/or via

	Yes	Somewhat	No	Comments
B.3. Multiple-choice examinations?				
B.4. Written dissertation?				
B.5. Examination of a patient interview (using video)?				
B.6. Medical record audits?				
B.7. Other?				
C. Are the residents given sufficient responsibility for their caseload, commensurate with their level of training, in:				
C.1. Clinical care?				
C.2. Clinical–administrative care?				
2. A. Do the supervisors know what is expected of them—for example, by means of:				
A.1. Knowing what level of skill the resident is expected to achieve in certain given areas as per lists of objectives?				
A.2. Workshops or other forms of formal discussion and communication?				
B. Are the supervisors receiving adequate feedback—for example:				
B.1. Via residents' written evaluations?				
B.2. From peer review?				
3. A. Do the seminar leaders know what is expected of them—for example:				
A.1. By means of having a set of objectives for their section of the seminar series?				
A.2. By understanding how their section fits into the total academic program (total set of cognitive learning objectives)?				
A.3. By discussion with the section leader and other staff involved in their seminar module?				
B. Are the seminar leaders receiving adequate feedback—for example, via residents' written evaluations?				
4. A. Are all academic or cognitive areas of psychiatric knowledge covered adequately (i.e., goals and objectives marked "essential" in Chapter 1*)—for example, by:				
A.1. Objectives with references?				

*No program will teach all areas equally well. Constructive comments on areas requiring improvement are important here.

	Yes	Somewhat	No	Comments
A.2. Lectures and seminars?				
A.3. Journal clubs?				
A.4. Visiting lecturers?				
A.5. Workshops?				
A.6. Support for attendance at out-of-town workshops?				
A.7. Other?				
B. With respect to the didactic programs, are faculty and residents clear as to their:				
B.1. Emphasis?				
B.2. Breadth?				
B.3. Depth?				
B.4. Quality?				
5. Are all skill areas necessary for the knowledgeable, safe, sound practice of psychiatry sufficiently taught and supervised (i.e., can and do residents complete under adequate supervision all tasks listed in the log book*) —for example, by:				
5.1. Direct supervision (supervisor present at some of the interviews)?				
5.2. Group supervision?				
5.3. Review of videotaped sessions?				
5.4. Audit of patient care and medical records?				
5.5. Supervision of their supervision of more junior colleagues and other mental health workers?				
5.6. Critical review of their case conference presentations?				
5.7. Other?				
6. Are the residents receiving sufficient exposure to all the areas of psychiatric practice (i.e., are they exposed to all types of patients and practice listed in the log book)—for example:				
6.1. Psychoses?				
6.2. "Neuroses"?				

*No program will teach all areas equally well. Constructive comments on areas requiring improvement are important here.

	Yes	Somewhat	No	Comments
6.3. Personality disorders? in different settings with patients with a wide variety of demographic characteristics?				
7. Is there adequate opportunity for collaboration with other mental health disciplines (see the log book)?				
8. Are the residents receiving adequate exposure to other community groups or agencies who are involved in the delivery of human services (see the log book)?				
9. Does the resident's service load infringe unduly on his other educational activities?				
10. With respect to research, do the residents have sufficient opportunity to:				
10.1. Learn how to critically evaluate scientific literature?				
10.2. Participate in clinical or basic research projects?				
11. Do the residents and staff both maintain a critical attitude toward both the program and the field as a whole?				
12. Do the residents have opportunities to get to know faculty members informally, during working hours and socially?				
13. Can residents obtain adequate and appropriate assistance for personal and professional problems and advice in career selection?				
14. Notwithstanding all the foregoing, are the residents sufficiently involved in ongoing self-monitoring and self-assessment?				

Section IV. Outcome
(Optional)

	Yes	Somewhat	No	
1. Has the program produced knowledgeable and skillful psychiatric specialists?				
1.1. In-program evaluations				
1.1.1. Skill				
a. Results of records and treatment outcome audits				

	Yes	Somewhat	No	Comments
b. Results of examinations of patient interview techniques (e.g., with examiner in room using standardized rating scale)				
c. Results of standardized tests using pretaped patient interviews				
1.1.2. Knowledge				
a. Multiple-choice exam results				
b. Dissertation results (where applicable)				
1.2. Termination evaluation				
1.2.1. Board or college examination results				
1.2.2. Follow-up evaluations: Survey of graduates' professional activities				
1.2.3. Outcome of the condition of patients who have been treated by trainees				
2. Has the program contributed significantly to other training programs—for example:				
2.1. Family medicine?				
2.2. Medical students?				
2.3. Other disciplines?				
3. Has the program contributed to the continuing education of:				
3.1. Psychiatrists?				
3.2. Other physicians?				
3.3. Other disciplines?				
3.4. The public?				
3.5. The government?				

ACKNOWLEDGMENT

To my residents, who forced me to evaluate.

Chapter 4   *by Peter B. Henderson*

Terminal and Enabling Objectives for Residency Training in Child Psychiatry

Foreword: Child Psychiatry Specialist Training

This chapter represents an experiment within the framework of developing educational objectives for subspecialty areas in psychiatric residency training. It was, however, requested later in the process of the development of this guide, and therefore could not go through the same series of reviews and discussions as the remainder of the material. The aim was to take an area of specialization in psychiatry and, by applying the same criteria of terminal and enabling objectives, see how this approach would fit with the field. As presented, it must be read in conjunction with the totality of the material in Chapter 1. Were it a free-standing section, it would present a more comprehensive picture than it does as an addendum to the overall material. Thus, to optimize one's use of this material, one must realize that it constitutes additions to and slight revisions of the earlier material, and those earlier sections must be referred to when studying these child psychiatry objectives.

    This method of presenting additional material could leave the impression, although it is not the intention to do so, that child psychiatry is merely an add-on to adult psychiatric training. It would be unfortunate if this were the conclusion derived, since this would be an unfair reflection of the field of child psychiatry. Basically, the difference between these two major areas of the psychiatric field is

Peter B. Henderson, M.D. • Associate Professor and Director of Residency Training in General and Child Psychiatry, University of Pittsburgh School of Medicine; Chairman, Committee on Training, American Academy of Child Psychiatry; Senior Editor, "The Basic Essentials of Training and Education of the Child Psychiatrist."

the matter of emphasis, practice, and application of knowledge and methods of necessary conduct of clinical work. The basic differences, and these should be kept in mind in reading this section, are:

1. The child is a dependent organism. An approach to the child in isolation is therefore rarely effective in either diagnostic or therapeutic work. The unit of concern is the ecological unit—that is, the child within his family within the context of the society and the various agencies that affect and can aid the child indirectly as well as directly. It may be possible to treat the adult effectively with little reference to family, the work place, or the social contacts. It is impossible to understand and treat the problems of children, however, without considering the context of the family and the forces that lead to its functioning, effectively or ineffectively, in its child-rearing role.
2. The child is a developing organism. This introduces an additional axis of consideration—namely, the age and stage at which the child presents as having problems. Thus, not only must one judge the normality or deviance of behavior, but also one must simultaneously relate this to the child's developmental stage, the tasks, and "the normal symptoms for that stage." To illustrate, the approach to temper tantrums in a three-year-old, an age at which tantrums are almost an expected part of the scene, is a very different approach than is used with the same problem at the age of ten.
3. The language of children is action and play, rather than verbalization. Comfort with and ability to use this mode of communication both for gathering information and for treating the child is a skill that can be developed only by experience, but without it the approach to many children is impossible.
4. The treatment of children requires a team approach. A significant difference commented on regularly by practitioners and by residents is the different function and role of the diagnostic and treating team. While teamwork can become time-consuming, inefficient, and a process of consensual validation of tenuously based conclusions, nevertheless, to handle adequately the majority of situations presented by children, the team that brings different skills to bear on the problem is essential for complete review, adequate assessment, and therapy. The team can be ancillary in many adult situations; in child psychiatry, it is central. This is not to imply that decisions are always made by mutual agreement, but more than the skills are complementary. Each skill is necessary but not alone sufficient.

The differences in the training requirements for the child psychiatry specialist are thus not only in the data base with its considerably greater depth in the areas discussed above, but also in the application of a unique method of case management.

The additional enabling objectives included in this chapter attempt to address these differences between adult and child psychiatry, which are more of emphasis than simply of knowledge. The danger, however, in addressing this problem by simply listing objectives as done in this chapter is that the essential overriding differences in emphasis, as noted above, can be lost in the detail.

Finally, and it is a caveat in general, reference lists for resident usage tend in all countries to have a peculiarly parochial slant—in Britain, from largely British literature; in North American literature, from North American journals. While a few lists straddle this geographic gap, it is repeatedly obvious that the synthesis of other than a small number of very classic papers from different countries is an issue that continually has to be addressed and, even where reading lists may only be guides, kept up to date.

The purpose of this introduction is therefore to underline both the essential similarities and the important differences between child and adult psychiatry. It is hoped that this chapter will go some way toward achieving perspective while maintaining an awareness that the differences are not polarities but are aspects of orientation and practice so that the child psychiatrist is appropriately equipped to handle effectively those situations with children and their families that the general psychiatrist rightly judges to be beyond his area of competence, desire, interest, or practice pattern.

Quentin Rae-Grant, M.D.

Professor and Vice-Chairman
University of Toronto

Psychiatrist-in-Chief
Hospital for Sick Children
Toronto, Ontario, Canada

Introduction

This chapter was prepared in collaboration with the editor. It arises from the primary author's work on "The Basic Essentials of Training and Education of the Child Psychiatrist," which is being prepared with input contributed by members of the American Academy of Child Psychiatry's Committee on Training. This document is one that has been nearly three years in preparation. Each re-edition of this document has followed a national survey and discussion at the Annual Meeting of the American Academy of Child Psychiatry.

It appeared obvious in reviewing the questionnaire following each of these national surveys, plus input from the Academy Committee on Training and from other members of the American Academy of Child Psychiatry who have been asked to contribute, that the generic issues of the basic "generalist" psychiatry core are also a rudimentary and fundamental part of the training of child psychiatrists. Certainly, however, there are distinctions, differences, and additions to the basic core curriculum that must be mastered to become a child psychiatrist (and therefore, in the United States, eligible for both general and child psychiatry board certification by the American Board of Psychiatry and Neurology).

The following pages are therefore designed to supplement and expand Chapter 1 with respect to the training of the subspecialist in child psychiatry. It is significant to note that no deletions of objectives written in Chapter 1 were considered necessary in this edited supplement; instead, the subspecialist in child psychiatry is anticipated to have mastered the core essentials in Chapter 1 and then to go into greater depth and a wider scope of study in the twenty basic areas as they relate specifically to the practice of psychiatry with children, adolescents, and their families.

The basic stylistic format and outline of the original manual have been preserved throughout this chapter. As with Chapter 1, the following pages are not meant to be a textbook or a syllabus.

In supplementing Chapter 1, all the "objectives" are listed in the same order as they are in Chapter 1. To further minimize redundancy and to maintain standardization of format, frequent reference will be made to the original twenty major areas and subdivisions thereof as follows:

> The upper case Roman numerals I through XX designate the twenty major sections into which this chapter is divided (see Fig. 1 on p. 4).
>
> Upper case letters A, B, C, etc., designate the topics (if any) into which a section is divided.
>
> Lower case Roman numerals i, ii, iii, etc., designate the subtopics (if any) into which a topic is divided.
>
> The subdivisions (if any) of each section are listed under the heading GENERAL PLAN.
>
> For a given section, topic, or subtopic, as appropriate, there is a statement of one or more TERMINAL OBJECTIVES.
>
> Under each subdivision is a list of ENABLING OBJECTIVES, plus more specific content-oriented "guides" (including bibliographic citations). Arabic numerals 1, 2, 3, etc., designate these enabling objectives; subdivisions are designated by 1.1, 1.2, 1.3, etc., and further subdivisions, where necessary, by 1.1.1, 1.1.2, 1.1.3, etc. Lower case letters a, b, c, etc., designate aspects of a given enabling objective (or subdivision thereof) to which attention should be given.

It should also be noted that:

1. All lists of objectives and subdivisions thereof are open-ended, it being assumed that future additions will be made as the subject areas of knowledge and skill are expanded within the different areas of the field of psychiatry.

2. The bibliographic citations should be added to, deleted, or in other ways modified in the future. These citations reflect the content areas considered necessary for addition to the basic guide, and are identified by authors' names and the year of publication.

3. As with Chapter 1, the listing of bibliographic citations and particular authors' names is not intended to force the resident in psychiatry to learn that particular work. These citations, as in the original guide, are simply guides to the subject areas referenced.*

---

*Liberal reference has been made to those core bibliographic references that were selected by Irving N. Berlin, M.D., senior editor of *A Bibliography of Child Psychiatry and Child Mental Health* (a monograph of the *Journal of the American Academy of Child Psychiatry*). The bibliography offers a reading list for all training program directors and a comprehensive set of references for those who wish to go deeper and wider into the literature on a specific topic. However, those references that were edited from the bibliography for inclusion in this text are considered by Dr. Berlin and his collaborators to be the most frequently referenced and significant literature citations in the child psychiatric educational endeavors in the United States (Berlin, 1976). The guides at the end of each subtopic contain authors' names and publication dates. These correspond to books and articles in the bibliography

4. Topics such as personality theories, neurotic disorders, and the treatment of the neuroses are certainly interrelated subjects. For purposes of specificity in outlining educational objectives, however, they are treated separately but cross-referenced.

5. Many of the same objectives as would be found, for example, under the general section on personality theories relate equally well to the understanding of the corresponding section in child and adolescent psychiatry. Objectives have therefore *not* been rewritten. It is understood that the resident who is specializing in child psychiatry will review all the objectives in Chapter 1 from the point of view of understanding and treating the child and his/her family. This process will, of course, somewhat alter the priority weighting given to particular objectives in Chapter 1. Statements as to high and low emphasis have not, for the most part, been given in this chapter, and it is the editor's hope that this ranking will be done in the individual training centers.

Section I.   Historical Trends in Child Psychiatry

TERMINAL OBJECTIVE

To understand the significance of psychiatry and child psychiatry in modern clinical practice and research.

ENABLING OBJECTIVES

1-3. See Chapter 1.
4. Be able to discuss the major trends in contemporary child psychiatry.

Guide: Include:
4.1–4.3. See Chapter 1.
4.4. Contributions of child psychiatry——This should include the original evolution of the child guidance clinic from the juvenile court and welfare system (Axelrod, 1955), as well as the movement from a subspecialty area that has been dominated by clinical practice to one that has taken major strides in the areas of research, community, and social interventions, and participated with the body of the psychiatric specialty in probing the basic science foundations of child psychiatry, child development, and developmental psychopathology.
4.5–4.7. See Chapter 1.
4.8. . . .
4.9. . . .
5-7. See Chapter 1.
8. . . .
9. . . .

---

at the end of the chapter. Again, they are given solely to help the resident begin his or her reading in this subspecialty and are *not* to be considered as lists of authors whose names or work should be committed to memory.

Section II.   Normality and Normal Psychosexual Development

GENERAL PLAN

A. Concept of Normality
B. Normal Psychosexual Development

TERMINAL OBJECTIVE

To be able to understand the importance of the concept of "normality" in child psychiatry.

A. Concept of Normality

ENABLING OBJECTIVES

1–3. See Chapter 1.
4. Be able to apply concepts derived from direct observations of normality to the clinical care of children and their families.

> *Guide:* Longitudinal studies and critical reformulations made by child developmentalists: Rexford (1969), Erikson (1959, 1963*a,b*), Freud, A. (1946), the Joint Commission on Mental Health of Children (infancy through adolescence) (1973).

5. . . .
6. . . .

B. Normal Psychosexual Development

TERMINAL OBJECTIVE

To know the psychological and-physiological aspects of normal sexual behavior and its development through different phases of life from infancy to maturity and old age.

ENABLING OBJECTIVES

1. See Chapter 1.
2. See Chapter 1. In addition to an understanding of the importance of psychosexual factors to clinical psychiatry, the child psychiatrist must be able to state and describe the ongoing, in-process elements of child development as they pertain to clinical interventions during the childhood and adolescent periods of the life cycle.

> *Guide:* References: Allen, F. H. (1963), Benedek (1970*a,b*), Erikson (1959), Freud, A. (1966*a,b*), Freud, S. (1953*a,b*), Rutter, M. (1971).

3. With respect to both the child and significant others in his environment, the child psychiatrist should be able to state the effect of:
a. Physical disabilities

b. *Physical illnesses*
c. *Medications*
d. ...
e. ...
on:
3.1. Gender and sexual identity
3.2. Role formation
3.3. Self-esteem
3.4. ...
3.5. ...

Guide: References: Prugh *et al.* (1953), Shrand (1965), Solnit (1960).

4. *Be able to compare and contrast male and female life cycle development, with major emphasis on resolution of crises and dilemmas pertaining to achievement, autonomy, motivation, affiliation, sexual identity, feminine and masculine role development, emancipation from the nuclear family, work motivation, marriage, etc.*
   4.1. See also Chapter 1, Section XIX.A, objective 5 (high emphasis).
   4.2. ...
   4.3. ...
5. ...
6. ...

Guide: References: Benedek, T. (1970*a,b*), Biller (1968), Deutsch, C. P. (1973), Greenbaum (1973). Group for the Advancement of Psychiatry: Committee on Public Education (1973).

Section III.   Contributions of the Biological Sciences to Psychiatry

(See Chapter 1, Introduction: Changes in the Delivery of Mental Health Care.)

GENERAL PLAN

A. Core Knowledge in Neuropsychiatry
B. Core Knowledge in Neuroendocrinology
C. Core Knowledge in Neurochemistry and Neurophysiology and the Relationship of These Sciences to Psychiatric Disorders
D. Memory
E. Sleep and Dreams
F. Experimental Psychopathology
G. Specialized Tests in Neurological Investigation
H. Neurological Correlates of Specialized Disorders

TERMINAL OBJECTIVE

To gain an understanding of the basic genetic, neurophysiological, and neurochemical mechanisms underlying behavior.

A. Core Knowledge in Neuropsychiatry

ENABLING OBJECTIVES

1. See Chapter 1.
2. See Chapter 1 and revise:
   2.1–2.4. See Chapter 1.
   2.5. The endocrine–autonomic nervous system–hypothalamus functions and their pathology.

   Guide: This should include drinking, eating, temperature regulation, sexual activity, and preparation for fight/flight. The child psychiatrist should be particularly cognizant of what these neuroendocrine functions (and potential dysfunctions) may produce in the evolving and growing organism of the immature child and young adolescent. References: Berkowitz (1961), Fish (1959).

   2.6. See Chapter 1.
   2.7. . . .
   2.8. . . .
3. . . .
4. . . .

B. Core Knowledge in Neuroendocrinology

ENABLING OBJECTIVES

1–4. See Chapter 1.
5. Be able to relate objectives 1–4 in Chapter 1 to the significance such findings may have in child liaison psychiatry.

   Guide: Emphasize endocrine disorders in children, and the impact of these disorders on the child's parents and surrounding environment. References: Book *et al.* (1963), Heeley and Roberts (1965).
6. . . .
7. . . .

C. Core Knowledge In Neurochemistry and Neurophysiology and the Relationship of These Sciences to Psychiatric Disorders

   No additions to enabling objectives listed in Chapter 1.

D. Memory

   No additions to enabling objectives listed in Chapter 1.

E. Sleep and Dreams

ENABLING OBJECTIVES

1-2. See Chapter 1.
3. In addition to being able to classify and describe major sleep disorders associated with psychiatric conditions, be able to outline changes in biological rhythms and individual variations in sleep physiology from infancy to adulthood.

> *Guide:* References: Anders and Weinstein (1973), Nagera (1964), Sperling (1955, 1958).

4-5. See Chapter 1.
6. . . .
7. . . .

F. Experimental Psychopathology

No additions to enabling objectives listed in Chapter 1.

G. Specialized Tests in Neurological Investigation

No additions to enabling objectives listed in Chapter 1.

H. Neurological Correlates of Specialized Procedures

No additions to enabling objectives listed in Chapter 1.

Section IV. Contributions of the Psychological Sciences to Psychiatry

GENERAL PLAN

A. Motivation
B. Ethology
C. Cognition
   i. Intelligence
   ii. Language Development
D. Perception
E. General Systems Theory
F. Communications Theory

TERMINAL OBJECTIVE

To be capable of applying knowledge and understanding of psychological research concepts and findings to clinical assessment, diagnostic formulation, and therapeutic management.

A. Motivation

No additions to enabling objectives listed in Chapter 1.

B. Ethology

ENABLING OBJECTIVES

1. *Be able to state the most outstanding contributions of the literature on ethology to our understanding of child development and human behavior.*

    Guide: References:
    Von Perneau (species-specific behavior)
    Lorenz (innate releasing mechanism, imprinting, action-specific energy)
    Tinbergen (displacement activity, hierarchy of appetitive behavior, and consumatory acts)
    Hess (imprinting)
    Von Holst and others on the neurophysiological basis of inborn behavior patterns
    Bowlby (infant behavior)
    Umwelt

2-4. See Chapter 1.
5. . . .
6. . . .

C. Cognition

Note: The following subtopics may be subsumed under the topic "cognition":
 i. Intelligence
 ii. Language Development
iii. Learning
iv. Memory
 v. Motivation
vi. Perception
All but i and ii are dealt with in other sections.

i. Intelligence (Thinking and Problem-Solving)

ENABLING OBJECTIVES

1. *See Chapter 1.*
2. *Be able to discuss, both with respect to general intelligence and with respect to specific factors in intelligence:*
    2.1-2.2. See Chapter 1.
    2.3. The relationship between intelligence and concept formation and "functional" mental disorders, e.g., schizophrenia, manic–depressive psychosis

    Guide: The child psychiatrist must also understand the cognitive components of learning disabilities, pseudoretardation and mental illness, and generalized underperformance in intellectual areas related to mental and behavioral disorders. References: Birch (1974), Jensen (1970), Thomas *et al.* (1961), Wolf (1965), Wolff (1970).

2.4. See Chapter 1.

2.5. . . .

2.6. . . .

3. See Chapter 1 and add:

Guide:

3.6. Illinois Test of Psycholinguistic Ability

3.7. Slingerland Reading and Language Disabilities Assessment

3.8. . . .

3.9. . . .

Reference: Douglas and Mulligan (1961)

4. See Chapter 1.

5. . . .

6. . . .

ii. Language Development

No additions to enabling objectives listed in Chapter 1.

D. Perception

ENABLING OBJECTIVES

1. See Chapter 1.

2. See Chapter 1 and note the addition to subobjective 2.2:

Guide:

2.1. See Chapter 1.

2.2. With respect to a clinical case, the child psychiatrist should be particularly attuned to the evolution of perceptual systems to include the "family perceptive system" and the relative differences between individual family members (note especially the effect of developmental level). References: Shapiro *et al.* (1972), Vernon (1965).

3-7. See Chapter 1.

8. . . .

9. . . .

E. General Systems Theory

ENABLING OBJECTIVES

1-3. See Chapter 1.

4. See Chapter 1 and add:

　　4.6. Understanding the interaction of endogenous and exogenous biopsychosocial factors in childhood development

Guide: Reference: Riskin and Faunce (1972).
4.7. . . .
4.8. . . .
5. . . .
6. . . .

F. Communications Theory

No additions to enabling objectives listed in Chapter 1.

Section V. Contributions of the Sociocultural Sciences to Psychiatry

GENERAL PLAN

A. Cultural Anthropology
    i. The Concept of Culture and Cultural Relativity
    ii. Cultural Variations in Marital Patterns and Family Structure
    iii. Cultural Change and Mental Health
B. Sociology, Ecology, and Social Psychiatry
    i. Concepts and Definitions
    ii. Social Class and Psychiatry
    iii. Important Ecological Factors Related to Psychiatric Disorders
    iv. The Sociology of Psychiatric Wards
C. Transcultural Psychiatry
    i. Variations in the Forms of Psychiatric Disorders According to Culture
    ii. Variations in the Epidemiology of Psychiatric Disorders According to Culture

A. Cultural Anthropology

i. The Concept of Culture and Cultural Relativity

No additions to terminal objective and enabling objectives listed in Chapter 1.

ii. Cultural Variations in Marital Patterns and Family Structure

TERMINAL OBJECTIVE

To learn the range and diversity of marital and family patterns across cultures and the ecological forces that may determine them.

ENABLING OBJECTIVES

1–4. See Chapter 1.
5. Be able to summarize how the cultural variations in family structure described

in objectives 1–4 above affect child and adolescent developmental stages and phases.

> *Guide:* References: Bronfenbrenner (1958, 1961), Emmerich (1968), Hess, R. D. (1970), Hess, R. D., and Shipman (1965). LeVine (1970), Lewis, O. (1959). McNickle (1968). Noshpitz (1970).

6. . . .
7. . . .

iii. Cultural Change and Mental Health

No additions to terminal objective and enabling objectives listed in Chapter 1.

B. Sociology, Ecology, and Social Psychiatry

i. Concepts and Definitions

TERMINAL OBJECTIVE

To become familiar with some of the main concepts and terms used by sociology when considering psychiatric phenomena.

ENABLING OBJECTIVES

1–3. See Chapter 1.
4. Be able to describe, using clinical case examples, interactions between role conflicts and parenting behavior(s).

> *Guide:* References: Clausen (1966), Kamii and Radin (1967). Lytton (1971), Miller, L. (1969).

5. . . .
6. . . .

ii. Social Class and Psychiatry

TERMINAL OBJECTIVE

To attain an understanding of what is meant by social class and how social class position may be related to psychiatric disorders, psychiatric treatment, and the attitudes of the psychiatrist.

ENABLING OBJECTIVES

1–4. See Chapter 1.
5. Be able to relate school and learning disorders, and problems in general achievement in children and adolescents, to problems related to their social class(es) (where applicable).

Guide: References: Harris and Roberts (1972), Hetznecker and Forman (1971), Malone (1967), Minuchin, S., and Montalvo (1967), Minuchin, P. P., *et al* (1969).

6. . . .
7. . . .

iii. Important Ecological Factors Related to Psychiatric Disorders

TERMINAL OBJECTIVE

To become familiar with research findings concerning relationships between various ecological factors and differential rates (and patterns) of psychiatric disorders.

ENABLING OBJECTIVES

1. See Chapter 1 and add:
   Guide:
   1.3. Be able to relate, in the clinical setting, factors in rural and urban schools that influence the incidence, prevalence. and patterns of learning disability and dysfunction. References: Birch and Gussow (1970), Chan *et al.* (1970), Karpman *et al.* (1952). Redl and Wineman (1951).
   1.4. . . .
   1.5. . . .
2. See Chapter 1.
3. . . .
4. . . .

iv. The Sociology of Psychiatric Wards

No additions to terminal objective and enabling objectives listed in Chapter 1.

C. Transcultural Psychiatry

No additions to the subtopics, terminal objectives, and enabling objectives listed in Chapter 1.

Section VI. Child and Adolescent Psychiatry

GENERAL PLAN

A. Child Psychiatry
   i. Child Development
   ii. Syndromes in Child Psychiatry
   iii. Treatment in Child Psychiatry
   iv. Adolescence and Its Problems
   v. Psychiatric Problems of the Child and Family

B. Mental Retardation
C. Genetics

A. Child Psychiatry

i. Child Development

TERMINAL OBJECTIVE

To become familiar with the major theories of child development, commencing with theories of attachment and preparation for child-rearing (relative to the pregnancy period) and extending through the major phases and subphases of human development throughout the life cycle. Major cognitive, psychosocial, psychosexual, growth, and maturational theories should be specifically mastered around developmental issues relevant to childhood, adolescence, and youth.

ENABLING OBJECTIVES

1-2. See Chapter 1.
3. See Chapter 1 and add:

> *Guide:* Child psychiatrists should note that most of these major conceptual frameworks do not sufficiently emphasize the developmental adaptations and maladaptations of the pregnancy period (with the exception of certain ego-psychologists who study carefully the theories of attachment and symbiosis during pregnancy). References: Benedek (1970*a,b*). Bibring *et al.* (1961), Jessner *et al.* (1970), Loesch and Greenberg (1962), Scheibel and Scheibel (1964), Winnicott (1965).

4. See Chapter 1.
5. . . .
6. . . .

ii. Syndromes in Child Psychiatry

TERMINAL OBJECTIVE

To become familiar with the major psychiatric syndromes encountered in children and adolescents, and how similar psychopathological syndromes may appear differently when presenting at different ages and developmental stages.

ENABLING OBJECTIVES

1. See Chapter 1 and add:

> *Guide:* References: Agras (1959), Berlin and Szurek (1965), Cytryn and McKnew (1974), Glaser (1967), Pearson (1952), Ric (1966), Rubenstein *et al.* (1959).

2. See Chapter 1.

3. See Chapter 1 and add:

Guide:
3.5.   Eisenberg, L.
3.6.   Rank, B.
3.7.   Rimland, B.
3.8.   Fish, B.
3.9.   . . .
3.10. . . .
4. . . .
5. . . .

iii. Treatment in Child Psychiatry

TERMINAL OBJECTIVES

1. To become familiar with the major forms of therapeutic intervention currently available within the field of child psychiatry, and to become proficient in at least two or three of the major interventions (e.g., child psychotherapy, family psychotherapy, group therapy with parents, chemotherapy).
2. To become expert in the selective use in differential treatment planning of each of the forms of treatment that can be soundly distinguished.

ENABLING OBJECTIVES

1. See Chapter 1 and add:
    1.8.   Play therapy and preschool and school-aged children
    1.9.   Sibling therapy

    Guide: References: White *et al.* (1972), Woltmann (1964).
    1.10.   . . .
    1.11.   . . .
2. See Chapter 1.
3. . . .
4. . . .
    Additional enabling objectives and subitems of experience are included under the individual treatment modalities in Section XVI.

iv. Adolescence and Its Problems

TERMINAL OBJECTIVES

To achieve an understanding of adolescence as a developmental stage, and to apply this understanding to an understanding of the psychopathology of adolescence.

ENABLING OBJECTIVES

1–5. See Chapter 1.
6. Be able to discuss several major contributors' theoretical approaches to adolescent development.

Guide: References: Berman (1970), Blos (1967), Erikson (1956), Group for the Advancement of Psychiatry: Committee on Adolescence (1968), Offer and Offer (1971).

7. . . .
8. . . .

v. Psychiatric Problems of the Child and Family*

TERMINAL OBJECTIVE

To understand disturbance in a child as it affects and is affected by the equilibrium of the family system.

ENABLING OBJECTIVES

1. See Chapter 1.
2. See Chapter 1 and add:
   2.9. The concept of generational boundaries
   2.10. The concept of multigenerational transmission systems
   2.11. . . .
   2.12. . . .
3. Be able to relate the child's developmental level to your decision to recommend or not recommend family therapy (in addition to, or instead of, other commonly available modalities).

   Guide: References: Boszormenyi-Nagy and Framo (1965), Bowen (1966), Fleck (1966), Jackson (1959), McDermott *et al.* (1976), Minuchin, S. (1965, 1974).
4. . . .
5. . . .

B. Mental Retardation

TERMINAL OBJECTIVE

To become aware that the problem of mental retardation involves the interplay of biological, psychological, social, and cultural factors, and that prevention and treatment must take account of this interplay.

ENABLING OBJECTIVES

1-4. See Chapter 1.
5. See Chapter 1 and note the changes in 5.1 and 5.2 and add 5.3:

   Guide:
   5.1. Discuss the biological, *genetic*, psychological, social, and cultural factors that may be involved and the interactions among them.
   5.2. *State and describe current knowledge concerning* the epidemiology of mental retardation.

---

*See also Section XVI.

5.3. Describe cases of mental retardation with no known or diagnosable etiology. References: Bender (1959), Eisenberg (1958a). Jakab (1970), Menolascino (1970). Valente and Tarjan (1974).

5.4. . . .

5.5. . . .

6. . . .

7. . . .

C. Genetics

No additions to terminal objective and enabling objectives listed in Chapter 1.

Section VII. Theories of Personality and Psychopathology

GENERAL PLAN

A. Personality Development and the Life Cycle
B. Personality Organization and Component Functions
C. Homeostasis, Motivation, Conflict, and Symptomatology
D. Phenomenology, Nosology, and General Psychopathology

TERMINAL OBJECTIVE

To be able to present an integrated theory of personality and its development, and to integrate the biological, psychological, and social components.

A. Personality Development and the Life Cycle

ENABLING OBJECTIVES

1-4. See Chapter 1.
5. Be thoroughly familiar with the work of Drs. R. Benedeck, M. Mahler, and D. Winnicott.
6. . . .
7. . . .

B. Personality Organization and Component Functions

ENABLING OBJECTIVES

1-7. See Chapter 1.
 8. See Chapter 1 and add:
  8.4. Sexuality of children (as both a conscious and an unconscious phenomenon)

  Guide: Include the relationship of sexuality to the child's personality and defense structure–organization. References: Erikson (1963a), Freud, S. (1953a,b), Kreitler and Kreitler (1966), Mead (1939), Schofield (1971).
  8.5. . . .
  8.6. . . .

9. . . .
10. . . .

C. Homeostasis, Motivation, Conflict, and Symptomatology

No additions to enabling objectives listed in Chapter 1.

D. Phenomenology, Nosology, and General Psychopathology

ENABLING OBJECTIVES

1. See Chapter 1.
   1.1. See Chapter 1.
   1.2. See Chapter 1 and add:

   Guide:
   1.2.10. Chess (Thomas and Chess, 1977)
   1.2.11. Freud, A. (1966a,b)
   1.2.12. Kessler (1971)
   1.2.13. Szurek (Szurek and Philips, 1973)
   1.2.14. . . .
   1.2.15. . . .
   1.3. See Chapter 1.
2. See Chapter 1.
3. . . .
4. . . .

Section VIII. Psychiatric Assessment

GENERAL PLAN

A. The Interview
B. Assessment in Psychiatry
C. Nosology

A. The Interview

TERMINAL OBJECTIVE

See Chapter 1.

ENABLING OBJECTIVES

1-10. See Chapter 1 and add:

   Guide: Emphasis on "developmental history" and on interviewing the child and his/her family.   Reference: Cohen *et al.* (1975).
11. . . .
12. . . .

B. Assessment in Psychiatry

TERMINAL OBJECTIVE

See Chapter 1 and revise as follows:

Guide:
1. Be able to evaluate children (demonstrating skills in applying interviewing techniques that are adapted to the developmental level of the child). It is particularly important that child psychiatric specialists be highly skilled in the use of play interviews, and in the understanding of verbal, nonverbal, play, and "body language" in the assessment of the child.
2. See Chapter 1.

ENABLING OBJECTIVES

No additions to enabling objectives listed in Chapter 1.

C. Nosology

TERMINAL OBJECTIVE

See Chapter 1.

ENABLING OBJECTIVES

1-4. See Chapter 1.
5. *Be able to discuss the implications of the newest nosological and classification systems, ICD-9 and DSM-III, particularly as they relate (or do not relate very well) to frequently seen children's psychopathological disorders.*

   Guide: References: Group for the Advancement of Psychiatry: Committee on Child Psychiatry (1966), Rutter *et al.* (1969), Miller, E. (1968), Fish and Shapiro (1965), Fish (1969), Szasz (1957), Freud, A. (1970).
6. . . .
7. . . .

Section IX. Psychiatric Emergencies and Reactive Disorders

GENERAL PLAN

A. Crisis Theory
B. Psychiatric Emergencies
C. Suicide
D. Transient Situational and Reactive Disorders
   i. Stress Reaction
   ii. Acute Grief Reaction

iii. Combat Neuroses
iv. Acute Culture-Bound Reactions
Add:
v. Marital Crisis

A. Crisis Theory

No additions to terminal objective or enabling objectives listed in Chapter 1.

B. Psychiatric Emergencies

TERMINAL OBJECTIVE

See Chapter 1.

ENABLING OBJECTIVES

1. See Chapter 1 and add:

Guide: In addition to subobjectives 1.1–1.15 in Chapter 1, the child subspecialist should have highly developed knowledge and experience in dealing with:
1.16. School phobia (acute)
1.17. School refusals (acute, particularly in adolescence)
1.18. Runaway behavior
1.19. Fire-setting
References: Johnson *et al.* (1941), Eisenberg (1958*b*), Hersov (1960), Vandersall and Weiner (1970), Howell *et al.* (1973).
1.20. . . .
1.21. . . .
2. . . .
3. . . .

C. Suicide

TERMINAL OBJECTIVE

See Chapter 1.

ENABLING OBJECTIVES

1–9. See Chapter 1.
10. Be able to relate knowledge and skills from objectives 1–9 above to suicide in children or young adolescents.

Guide: References: Ackerly (1967), Mattson (1969).
11. Be able to assess and manage the adverse effects of suicide by one family member on other members of his or her family.

12. ...
13. ...

D. Transient Situational and Reactive Disorders

Subtopics i–iv

No additions to terminal or enabling objectives listed in Chapter 1.

v. Marital Crisis

ENABLING OBJECTIVES

1. Be able, in the clinical setting, to recognize and describe:
    1.1. Acute vs. chronic marital disorder
    1.2. Effects on siblings of a symptomatic child
    1.3. Extent of marital disorder

    Guide: Generalized or specific to a single area (e.g., sex, family, money).
    1.4. Transfer of symptomatology from one sibling to another when a symptom-bearing child is removed from a crisis-influenced family setting
    1.5. ...
    1.6. ...
2. Be able to assess and treat the marital couple in crisis.

    Guide: References: Lidz (1961), Vogel (1960), Fleck (1966), Tseng *et al.* (1977), Nagera (1970).
3. ...
4. ...

Section X. Psyche and Soma and Liaison Psychiatry

TERMINAL OBJECTIVE

See Chapter 1.

ENABLING OBJECTIVES

1. See Chapter 1.
2. See Chapter 1 and add:
    2.5. Be able to state the effects of illness in one family member on:
        2.5.1. Other family members
        2.5.2. The family as a system (equilibrium)
        2.5.3. Significant others

    Guide: Include effects of disfigurement (stigma).
    2.6. ...
    2.7. ...

3. See Chapter 1 and add:

3.6. Be able to consult effectively with professional staff and family members with respect to evolving a treatment plan that includes the total family, considers all salient supportive dynamics, and focuses on the prevention of childhood developmental difficulties.

3.7. . . .

3.8. . . .

4. See Chapter 1 and add:

4.5. Be able to attune ward and clinic staff to the developmental needs of the child patient who is the consultee in a given clinical situation.

Guide: References: Schur (1955), Benedek (1949), Koupernik (1973), Szurek (1951), Offord and Aponte (1967), Green (1967), Schowalter and Solnit (1966).

4.6. . . .

4.7. . . .

5. . . .

6. . . .

Section XI.   The Neuroses, Personality Disorders, Addictions, and Sexual Disorders
—Including Disorders That Are Associated Primarily with Affective, Anxiety, "Somatoform," Dissociative, Factitious, Impulse-Control, Drug-Use, Psychosexual, and Personality Problems

GENERAL PLAN

A. The Neuroses
B. Personality Disorders
C. Drug-Use Disorders
D. Psychosexual Disorders

TERMINAL OBJECTIVE

On the basis of a broad knowledge of modern theories of etiology and the various treatment modalities and with knowledge of the limitations thereof, to be able to assess, formulate, diagnose, and treat the conditions discussed in this section.

GENERAL ENABLING OBJECTIVES APPLICABLE TO ALL
TOPICS

No additions to enabling objectives listed in Chapter 1.

SPECIFIC ENABLING OBJECTIVES APPLICABLE TO EACH
TOPIC

A. The Neuroses

1. See Chapter 1.
2. See Chapter 1 and add:

> *Guide:*
> 2.6. Include theories of neuroses developed from direct observations of parent–
> child interactions.
>
> *Guide:* References: Freud, A. (1966*a,b*), Nagera (1964), Anthony (1967),
> Sperling (1955), Rank *et al.* (1948).

2.7. . . .
2.8. . . .
3. See Chapter 1.
> 3.1. See Chapter 1 and add:
>
> > *Guide:* The child psychiatrist should be aware of the child's sensitivity to
> > drug interactions, particularly when managing physically ill children, very
> > young children, or children of labile temperament.
>
> 3.2. See Chapter 1 and add:
>
> > The use of appropriate psychotherapeutic measures—individual (*adult
> > and child interventions*), . . .
> >
> > *Guide:* References: Weiner (1977), Fish (1960, 1968), Grant (1962).
>
> 3.3–3.4. See Chapter 1.
> 3.5. . . .
> 3.6. . . .

4. See Chapter 1.
5. . . .
6. . . .

B. Personality Disorders

1. See Chapter 1.
> *1.1.–1.2. See Chapter 1.*
> *1.3. See Chapter 1 and add:*
> > *1.3.2. Chess, S., and Thomas, A.*
> > *1.3.3. Offer, D., and Offer, J.*
> > *1.3.4. . . .*
> > *1.3.5. . . .*
> *1.4. See Chapter 1 and add:*
> > *1.4.2. Dubos, R.*
> > *1.4.3. Hess, R. D.*
> > *1.4.4. . . .*
> > *1.4.5. . . .*

Guide: References: Thomas and Chess (1977), Offer and Offer (1971), Dubos (1968), Hess (1964).
  1.5. . . .
  1.6. . . .
2. *See Chapter 1 and add:*
  2.4. Use of individual therapy, individual treatment
  2.5. Family therapy of childhood and adolescent behavior disorders.

  Guide: See Section XVI.
  2.6. . . .
  2.7. . . .
3. *See Chapter 1 and add:*
  3.1. Be able to set realistic goals with the child patient when age and developmental level make this a reasonable possibility.
  3.2. Be able to formulate a goal-oriented treatment contract with the child's parent(s).

  Guide: References: Axelrod (1955), Karpman *et al.* (1952).
  3.3. . . .
  3.4. . . .
4. *See Chapter 1.*
5. . . .
6. . . .

C. Drug-Use Disorders (Including Alcoholism and Drug Dependencies)

1–7. See Chapter 1.
  8. *Be able to describe the effects of alcoholism in a family member on:*
  8.1. Other family members
  8.2. The family "system"

  Guide: References: Straus (1973), Paredes *et al.* (1973), Chafetz *et al.* (1971).
  9. . . .
10. . . .

D. Psychosexual Disorders

(In child psychiatry, this title should perhaps be "problems in sexual development.")
1. *See Chapter 1.*
2. *See Chapter 1 and add:*

  Guide:
  2.5. Marital and family therapy (particularly where a child's sexual behavior problems may be related to marital and/or family tension and conflict). References: Lewis, M., and Sarrel (1969), Harrison (1970), Johnson and Robinson (1957), Matza (1969).

2.6. . . .

2.7. . . .

3. *Be able to describe the familial factors that relate to deviant role assignments by parents and that may relate to the development of sexual identity distur-bances in children and adolescents, including:*

    3.1. Possible constitutional and genetic predisposing factors

    3.2. Unresolved familial alliances and pathological behaviors

    3.3. . . .

    3.4. . . .

4. *. . .*

5. *. . .*

Section XII. The "Functional" Psychoses

GENERAL PLAN

A. The Schizophrenic Disorders

B. Paranoid Disorders

C. Affective Disorders—Psychotic

D. "Borderline" States

E. Brief Reactive Disorders

F. Atypical "Psychoses"

G. Other Psychoses

Add:

H. Psychoses in Childhood

> *Guide:* Include:
>
> 1. Early childhood psychoses
>   a. Early infantile autism (Kanner, 1943)
>   b. Symbiotic psychosis (Mahler, 1952)
>   c. Children with atypical ego development (Rank and Kaplan, 1950)
> 2. Childhood schizophrenia
>   a. Process disorders (Goldfarb and Forsen, 1956)
>   b. Biological determinants (Rutter, 1972)
>   c. Familial factors (Lidz *et al.*, 1957; Lidz, 1958)
> 3. Other psychoses in children
>   a. "Borderline condition" (Ekstein and Wallerstein, 1956, 1957)
>   b. Manic–depressive disorders in childhood (Anthony and Scott, 1960)
>   c. Anaclitic depressions (with psychotic residual) (Spitz and Wolf, 1946)

TERMINAL OBJECTIVES

1. *See Chapter 1.*

2. To be able to interview, diagnose, and manage the treatment of patients *and their families.*

ENABLING OBJECTIVES APPLICABLE TO ALL FUNCTIONAL PSYCHOSES: GENERAL

1. See Chapter 1.
   1.1. See Chapter 1 and add:

      Guide:
      1.1.5.   Bender and Gureivitz (1955)
      1.1.6.   Bateson *et al.* (1956)
      1.1.7.   Mahler (1952, 1967)
      1.1.8.   Kanner (1943, 1944)
      1.1.9.   Eisenberg (1966)
      1.1.10. Szurek (1956)
      1.1.11. Bettelheim (1956)
      1.1.12. . . .
      1.1.13. . . .
   1.2–1.5. See Chapter 1.
   1.6. . . .
   1.7. . . .
2. See Chapter 1.
3. See Chapter 1.
   3.1. See Chapter 1.
   3.2. See Chapter 1.
      3.2.1–3.2.3. See Chapter 1.
      3.2.4. See Chapter 1 and add:

         Guide: References: Judd and Mandell (1968), Jackson (1960), Gregory (1960), Schain and Freedman (1961), Sankar *et al.* (1961), Hingtgen and Bryson (1974).

      3.2.5. . . .
      3.2.6. . . .
   3.3–3.6. See Chapter 1.
   3.7. . . .
   3.8. . . .
4–8. See Chapter 1.
9. . . .
10. . . .

ENABLING OBJECTIVES APPLICABLE TO ALL FUNCTIONAL PSYCHOSES: CLINICAL

1. Be able to demonstrate, by conducting clinical interviews with patients (in the case of child psychiatrists, the child patient and his/her family and significant others) suffering from major psychoses, the capacity to:
   1.1. Establish therapeutic relationships with the child and, where appropriate, other family member(s).
   1.2. Elicit a history from the child (if possible) and from the parents or other important informants.

    1.3. See Chapter 1.
    1.4. See Chapter 1.
        1.4.1. See Chapter 1.
        1.4.2. A treatment program tailored to the needs of both the child and the family

            Guide: In the case of a psychotic child, family, social, and dynamic factors must be included in the treatment plan. In the management of future decompensations of the child, be able to assist the parents in understanding and functioning as allies within the treatment plan (include the long-term dispositional arrangements). References: Szurek (1956), Berlin and Szurek (1973), Ekstein and Wallerstein (1957), Kempf (1964).

        1.4.3. . . .
        1.4.4. . . .
    1.5. . . .
    1.6. . . .
2. . . .
3. . . .

ENABLING OBJECTIVES APPLICABLE TO SPECIFIC FUNCTIONAL PSYCHOSES

A. The Schizophrenic Disorders

    General and clinical objectives as above.

B. Paranoid Disorders

    No additions to enabling objectives listed in Chapter 1.

C. Affective Disorders—Psychotic

1–3. See Chapter 1.
4. With respect to bipolar and unipolar affective disorders in early childhood, be able to:
4.1. State precursors.
4.2. Describe the clinical appearance.

    Guide: Reference: Anthony and Scott (1960).
4.3. . . .
4.4. . . .
5. . . .
6. . . .

D. "Borderline" States

    No additions to enabling objectives listed in Chapter 1.

E. Brief Reactive Disorders

No additions to enabling objectives listed in Chapter 1.

F. Atypical "Psychoses"

No additions to enabling objectives listed in Chapter 1.

G. Other Psychoses

No additions to enabling objectives listed in Chapter 1.

H. Psychoses in Childhood

General and clinical objectives as above.

Section XIII. The Organic Mental Disorders

TERMINAL OBJECTIVE

To be able to recognize the clinical syndromes that can arise from organic disturbance of brain function; have sufficient knowledge of neuroanatomy, physiology, and pathology to appreciate the factors underlying such states; and know the common physical conditions that may produce such states and be able to diagnose and treat them.

ENABLING OBJECTIVES

1. Be able to describe the normal aging process from earliest embryogenesis through the gross morphological and related changes of extreme aging.

   Guide: The child psychiatric resident should pay particular attention to the cognitive development of children and to neurobiological factors in central nervous system maturation.

2-5. See Chapter 1.

6. See Chapter 1 and add:

   6.11. Adult and child minimal neurological disorders

   Guide: Discernible only by "soft" neurological signs or found only by administration of highly sensitive neuropsychological tests for organicity. References on organic mental disorders in children: Cravioto (1968), DeHirsch (1970), Dubin and Dubin (1965), Gesell and Amatruda (1947), Piaget (1970), Vernon (1965), Walters and Parke (1963), Bender (1956), Graffagnino *et al.* (1968), Chess (1960), Chess and Thomas (1972), Werry *et al.* (1964), Wender (1971).

   6.12. . . .

   6.13. . . .

7. See Chapter 1.
8. . . .
9. . . .

Section XIV.   The Organic Therapies

GENERAL PLAN

A. Psychopharmacology
B. Convulsive Therapies
C. Psychosurgery
D. Miscellaneous and Little-Used Biological Treatments

A. Psychopharmacology

TERMINAL OBJECTIVE

To learn about the safe use of psychotropic medications with respect to the prevention and treatment of psychiatric disorders.

ENABLING OBJECTIVES

1-2. See Chapter 1.
3. See Chapter 1 and add:
   3.16. Interactive effects of psychoactive medication(s) on the immature and developing central nervous system of the child and young adolescent

   Guide: References: Weiner (1977), Millichap (1968), Annell (1969), Freeman (1970), Fish (1971).
   3.17. . . .
   3.18. . . .
4-8. See Chapter 1.
9. . . .
10. . . .

B. Convulsive Therapies

Not applicable.

C. Psychosurgery

D. Miscellaneous and Little-Used Biological Treatments

Note: Topics B–D are rarely considered in typical practice or research in child psychiatry. They should be included, however, in the basic knowledge and skill base from the child psychiatrist's earlier specialization in the field of basic general psychiatry.

Section XV. Learning Theory and Behavior Modification

GENERAL PLAN

A. Learning Theory
B. Behavior Modification

A. Learning Theory

TERMINAL OBJECTIVE

To acquire a working knowledge of learning theory as it applies to the understanding of personality development and psychiatric disorders.

ENABLING OBJECTIVES

1-4. See Chapter 1.
5. Be able to state the implications of learning theory in role formation, maintenance, and role change, particularly in the therapeutic situation.

> *Guide:* References: Penick *et al.* (1971), Schell and Adams (1968), Blatt (1957), Clement (1971), Andronico *et al.* (1967).

6. . . .
7. . . .

B. Behavior Modification

TERMINAL OBJECTIVE

To learn the effective and ethical application of the principles of learning in the treatment of psychiatric disorders.

ENABLING OBJECTIVES

1. See Chapter 1.
2. Under supervision, be able to:
  2.1-2.2. See Chapter 1.
  2.3. See Chapter 1 and add:

> *Guide:* In the event the patient is a child, a child psychiatrist should involve parental cooperation, understanding, and participation; evolve a working alliance; and integrate a component of parent education into the behavioral therapeutic technique that is being employed. References: Levine and Levine (1970), Reinhart (1970).

  2.4-2.5. See Chapter 1.
  2.6. . . .
  2.7. . . .

3. See Chapter 1.
4. ...
5. ...

Section XVI. The Psychotherapies

GENERAL PLAN

A. Individual Psychotherapy
B. Group Psychotherapy
C. Family Psychotherapy
D. Psychotherapy with Children
E. Milieu Therapy
F. Activity and Rehabilitation "Therapies"

TERMINAL OBJECTIVES

1–2. See Chapter 1.
3. To develop an appreciation, through experience, of one's abilities and difficulties in using such techniques. For child psychiatrists, it is important to have a particularly well developed skill and knowledge base of therapeutic work with young children and adolescents.
4–5. See Chapter 1.

ENABLING OBJECTIVES FOR ALL PSYCHOTHERAPIES

1. Be able to demonstrate a psychodynamic understanding of the psychotherapeutic relationship, how it is started, formed, and terminated, and how it may be disrupted.

    Guide: Particular emphasis should be placed on the disruptions in child therapy that may occur related to (a) the developmental level or (b) the child's parents (e.g., lack of commitment to therapy).

2. See Chapter 1.
3. Be able to correctly "prescribe" appropriate treatment(s) and set realistic goals for each of them.

    Guide: Pay special attention to variations among child, couple, family, and individual adult needs.

4. See Chapter 1.
5. Be able to demonstrate, in the clinical setting, an awareness of the effects on the therapeutic process of those biases in both the therapist and the patient that arise from cultural stereotypes of male and female behavior, and from adult/child expectations.
6. See Chapter 1 and add:

    Guide: References: Meeks (1971), Blos (1962), Mattsson (1970), Ginott (1968), Bell and Vogel (1968), Kysar (1968), Weinrott (1974), Cohen *et al.* (1961), Rae-Grant and Marcuse (1968).

7. . . .
8. . . .

A. Individual Psychotherapy

ENABLING OBJECTIVES APPLICABLE TO TREATMENT
MODELS IN GENERAL

1. Perceptual and conceptual skills: Be able to:
 1.1.–1.2. See Chapter 1.
 1.3. See Chapter 1 and add:
  1.3.4. Be able, as a therapist, to act in the role of educator–catalyst for the immature younger child or extremely concrete-thinking patient.

   Guide: In these instances, some "fund of knowledge about the world" is necessary to facilitate a psychotherapeutic transaction.
  1.3.5. . . .
  1.3.6. . . .
 1.4. . . .
 1.5. . . .
2. Executive skills: Be able to:
 2.1–2.7. See Chapter 1.
 2.8. Demonstrate a working knowledge of the fundamentals of play therapy.

   Guide: Utilize varying play techniques, media, and other expressive modalities in the elaboration of play themes. Reference: Henderson (1977).
 2.9. . . .
 2.10. . . .
3. See Chapter 1.
4. . . .
5. . . .

ENABLING OBJECTIVES APPLICABLE TO SPECIFIC
TREATMENT MODELS

No additions to enabling objectives listed in Chapter 1.

B. Group Psychotherapy

ENABLING OBJECTIVES APPLICABLE TO GROUP TREATMENT
APPROACHES IN GENERAL

1–5. See Chapter 1.
6. Be able to identify and describe approaches appropriate for different categories and ages of groups and types of patients.

 Guide: Activity group therapy is a particularly important modality for the child psychiatrist to understand and experience. Reference: Ginott (1968).

7. See Chapter 1.
8. . . .
9. . . .

ENABLING OBJECTIVES APPLICABLE TO SPECIFIC GROUP TREATMENT APPROACHES

No additions to enabling objectives listed in Chapter 1.

C. Family Psychotherapy

ENABLING OBJECTIVES

1-2. See Chapter 1.
3. See Chapter 1 and add:

> *Guide:*
> The child psychiatrist should emphasize the influences on family dynamics of:
> l. Different developmental levels of the children
> m. The developmental needs of adult-age parents who are pursuing adult developmental crises at the time of therapy
> n. . . .
> o. . . .

4. See Chapter 1 and add:

> *Guide:* References: Tseng *et al.* (1976), Bowen (1966), Jackson (1959), MacGregor *et al.* (1964), Ferber *et al.* (1972).

5. . . .
6. . . .

D. Psychotherapy with Children

ENABLING OBJECTIVES

1-3. See Chapter 1.
4. See Chapter 1 and add:

> *Guide:* Have a minimum of six to eight long-term experiences throughout the residency program with individual children representing a variety of ages and psychopathology. It is important for the child specialist to obtain expertise in the treatment of the preschool, school-age, early and late adolescent child and his/her family. It is equally important that the psychopathology represented by these children and adolescents at their different stages of development be distinctly different enough that the child trainee is exposed to the widest variety of child and adolescent psychopathological symptomatology. At least two of the child cases should be in intensive supervised play psychotherapy. Additionally, the resident must become proficient in the evaluation of appropriate cases for child psychotherapeutic modalities of treatment and therefore should comprehensively assess approximately a dozen more patients

in the course of a 2- to 4-year training experience. References: McDermott *et al.* (1976), Rabinovitch (1964), Koppitz (1968), Coppolillo (1969), Levy (1968), Axelrod (1955), Philips (1966), Gruenberg and Leighton (1965), Fleming (1967), Klerman (1965), Szurek and Berlin (1956).

5. . . .

6. . . .

E. Milieu Therapy

No additions to enabling objective listed in Chapter 1.

F. Activity and Rehabilitation "Therapies"

No additions to enabling objective listed in Chapter 1.

Section XVII. Community and Administrative Psychiatry

GENERAL PLAN

A. Historical Development and Definition
B. Basic Psychiatric Principles
    i. The Concept of Prevention
    ii. Continuity of Care
    iii. Large-Group Dynamics
    iv. Team Functioning
C. Basic Administrative Principles
    i. Regionalization
    ii. Systems Theory
    iii. Management
    iv. Audits of Patient Care
D. Methods of Intervention
E. Research

TERMINAL OBJECTIVE

See Chapter 1.

A. Historical Development and Definition

ENABLING OBJECTIVES

1. See Chapter 1.
2. See Chapter 1 and add:
   2.3. Political changes

> *Guide:* Be able to discuss the developments leading up to, and evolving since, the formation of the Joint Commission (United States) on the Mental Health of Children, or an equivalent sociopolitical phenomenon

where applicable. as it relates both to the development of new child mental health–mental retardation resources in the community and to the amalgamation or improved coordination of existing services.

2.4. ...
2.5. ...
3. See Chapter 1.
4. ...
5. ...

B. Basic Psychiatric Principles

i. The Concept of Prevention

ENABLING OBJECTIVES

1-3. See Chapter 1.
4. See Chapter 1 and add:

Guide:
4.5. Appropriate recreational, educational. and cultural-specific activities available for children. youth, adults. and the aged
4.6. Acculturating or socializing effects, or both. of the physical environment on the community's children and youth.
References: Rexford (1976), Lowrey (1955). Barhash *et al*.(1951). Witmer (1940), Eisenberg (1969). Cassell (1966), Monroe *et al*. (1967). Birch and Gussow (1970). Joint Commission on Mental Health of Children (1970), Chase 1971).
4.7. ...
4.8. ...
5. *Be able to review critically the effects of "institutionalization,"* with special emphasis on children and adolescents.

Guide:
a. Effects of early separation
b. Institutional adult role models for developing and maturing children
c. Loss of sense of family membership
d. Dependency supports.
e. Interventions in pathological peer groupings
f. Remedial and specialized education
g. "Contagion" effects
References: Behrens and Goldfarb (1958), Davids *et al.* (1968), Ekstein *et al.* (1959), Wolfensberger (1969), LaVietes *et al.* (1960), Redl (1959), Henry (1957), Konopka (1954).
h. ...
i. ...
6. See Chapter 1.
7. ...
8. ...

ii. Continuity of Care

ENABLING OBJECTIVES

1. Be able to discuss the principle of continuity of care from the point of view of:
  1.1. The child patient and his/her family
  1.2. The professional
  1.3. The health care administrator
2. . . .
3. . . .

iii. Large-Group Dynamics

No additions to enabling objectives listed in Chapter 1.

iv. Team Functioning

ENABLING OBJECTIVES

1. See Chapter 1.
2. Be able to discuss the advantages and disadvantages of the treatment team working primarily in the community from the point of view of:
  2.1. The child patient and his/her family

  Guide: Both as groups of patients and as individuals with unique needs.
  2.2. The professional

  Guide: Clinical and administrative; service, education, and research.
  2.3. The community

  Guide: Its responsiveness to the specialized needs of disadvantaged, disturbed, and/or retarded children (who either have been institutionalized or are in a postinstitution rehabilitation–resocialization experience).
  with respect to:
  a. Effectiveness, coordination, role diffusion
  b. Efficiency, cost benefit
  c. . . .
  d. . . .
  References: Freud, A., and Dann (1951), Williams (1961), Naughton (1957).
3. . . .
4. . . .

C. Basic Administrative Principles

i. Regionalization

TERMINAL OBJECTIVE

To be able to discuss the concept of regionalization as it pertains to the delivery of mental health and retardation services.

ENABLING OBJECTIVES

1. See Chapter 1.
2. See Chapter 1 and add:

   Guide:
   The child psychiatrist should be sensitive to the number of specialized educators, "developmental" specialties, child health care delivery specialists, etc.
3–4. See Chapter 1.
5. . . .
6. . . .

Subtopics ii–iv

No additions to enabling objectives listed in Chapter 1.

D. Methods of Intervention

No additions to enabling objectives listed in Chapter 1.

E. Research

ENABLING OBJECTIVES

1. Be able to outline the methods of investigation and the principal conclusions of epidemiological, sociological, and developmental research pertinent to community practice of child psychiatry, including:
   1.1. Research relevant to the prevalence of mental illness
   1.2. Research relevant to the relationship between:
      1.2.1–1.2.3. See Chapter 1.
      1.2.4. Mental illness as a psychosocial phenomenon and "illness resulting from an incapacitating psychotoxic society"
      1.2.5. Biological and biosocial phenomena and maturational–developmental factors of children and their families

      Guide: References: Philips (1966), Tarjan (1959), Berlin (1966, 1969), Group for the Advancement of Psychiatry: Committee on Child Psychiatry (1973), Chess (1972), Call (1963), Schuman (1968), Engel (1961), Lindemann (1944), Caplan *et al.* (1965).

      1.2.6. . . .
      1.2.7. . . .
   1.3. . . .
   1.4. . . .
2. . . .
3. . . .

Section XVIII. Geriatric and Forensic Psychiatry

GENERAL PLAN

A. Geriatric Psychiatry
B. Forensic Psychiatry
    i. Psychiatry and Criminal Law
    ii. The Concept of Competency
    iii. Compulsory Detention and Treatment, Where Applicable, of the Mentally Ill

A. Geriatric Psychiatry

TERMINAL OBJECTIVE

To learn how to evaluate, diagnose, and treat psychiatric illnesses in the geriatric age group.

ENABLING OBJECTIVES

1–7. See Chapter 1.
 8. This objective might be slightly revised to facilitate the education of the child psychiatrist, as follows:
  Using theoretical knowledge of biopsychosocial phenomenology and the process of mourning, one should be able to manage issues concerning death and dying in the clinical setting with respect to:
  8.1. The aged patient
  8.2. The family (including its youngest member)
  8.3. Other caretakers (e.g., ward nurses)
  8.4. Self

  Guide: References: Nolfi (1967), Kalish (1965).
 9. See Chapter 1.
10. . . .
11. . . .

B. Forensic Psychiatry

i. Psychiatry and Criminal Law

TERMINAL OBJECTIVE

To be cognizant of the relationship between criminal law and mental disorder (illness or retardation).

ENABLING OBJECTIVES

1-2. See Chapter 1.
  3. See Chapter 1 and add:
    3.3. Children to assume adversarial positions against parent(s) with full legal
       representation
    3.4. . . .
    3.5. . . .
  4-6. See Chapter 1.
  7. See Chapter 1 and add:
    7.4. Who, because of "tender age," can be placed under psychiatric observa-
       tion or care or both
    7.5. . . .
    7.6. . . .
  8. Be able to state and discuss the review procedures available for persons held
    involuntarily in psychiatric facilities, including the commitment procedures
    for adolescents and children, which (e.g., in some states in the United States)
    involve legal representation and changes in child civil liberties.

    Guide: Reference: Cheney (1966).
  9. Be able to state the legal procedures relevant to child custody cases in your
    state or province.
  10. Be able to:
    10.1. Write a document sufficient for presentation in a testimonial setting
       that would represent the child psychiatrist as the advocate of the child
       in a court proceeding.
    10.2. Function as the amicus curiae *of the judge (i.e., present psychiatric*
       findings from both the parental and child clinical evaluations that could
       be used as clinical data for court evidence).
    10.3. . . .
    10.4. . . .
11. . . .
12. . . .

ii. The Concept of Competency

TERMINAL OBJECTIVE

To examine the concept of competency in relationship to mental illness or retardation.

ENABLING OBJECTIVES

1. See Chapter 1 and add:
  1.7. Informed consent related to tender years
  1.8. . . .
  1.9. . . .

2. . . .
3. . . .

iii. Compulsory Detection and Treatment, Where Applicable, of the Mentally III

TERMINAL OBJECTIVE

To be familiar with the legislation governing the detention of the mentally disordered and retarded.

ENABLING OBJECTIVES

See Chapter 1 and add:

Guide: References: Curran (1968), Gil (1960), Westman and Cline (1971), Goldstein *et al.* (1970), Kleinfield (1971), Foster (1973), Proposed Revised Uniform Marriage and Divorce Act (1973), Mercer (1974), Rosenheim (1973).

Section XIX. Gender and Psychiatry

No additions to terminal and enabling objectives listed in Chapter 1. Those objectives that deal with child development are of particular importance.

Section XX. Psychiatric Research and Evaluation

GENERAL PLAN

A. History and Philosophy of Psychiatric Research Design
B. Models, Statistics, and Computers in Psychiatry
C. Psychiatric Epidemiology as Human Ecology
D. Evaluation of Psychiatric Treatment, Treatment Programs, and Training

A. History and Philosophy of Psychiatric Research Design

No additions to terminal objective listed in Chapter 1.

B. Models, Statistics, and Computers in Psychiatry

ENABLING OBJECTIVES

1. See Chapter 1 and add:

   Guide:
   1.8.   Developmental research and theories
   1.9.   Deprivation modes and models

1.10. . . .
1.11. . . .
2-6. See Chapter 1 and add:

   Guide: References: Escalona and Heider (1959), Kris (1957), Achenbach and Lewis (1971), Stennett (1966), Chess *et al.* (1967), Langner *et al.* (1970), Sze (1971).
7. . . .
8. . . .

C. Psychiatric Epidemiology as Human Ecology

ENABLING OBJECTIVES

1-6. These objectives are general in their application for the general psychiatrist or child psychiatrist. Subobjective 6.7 should also include a longitudinal-developmental perspective with respect to the child psychiatrist's ability to differentiate individual, familial, social, and ecological factors in the differential analysis of illness findings (e.g., statistics, raw data, derivations of deviance and disease).
7. . . .
8. . . .

D. Evaluation of Psychiatric Treatment, Treatment Programs, and Training

ENABLING OBJECTIVES

1-6. These objectives are generally applicable to both general and child psychiatrists.
7. Be able to constructively evaluate one's practice requirements and demonstrate active participation in formal and informal educative processes to maintain the level of competence required for one's regular professional activities.
8. See comment regarding objectives 1-6 above.
9. . . .
10. . . .

Bibliography

Achenbach, T. M., and Lewis, M. "A Proposed Model for Clinical Research and Its Application to Encopresis and Enuresis." *J. Am. Acad. Child Psychiatry* **10**:535–554, 1971.

Ackerly, W. C. "Latency-Age Children Who Threaten or Attempt to Kill Themselves." *J. Am. Acad. Child Psychiatry* **6**:242–261, 1967.

Agras, S. "The Relationship of School Phobia to Childhood Depression." *Am. J. Psychiatry* **116**:533–536, 1959.

Allen, F. H. "The Dilemma of Growth." In: *Positive Aspects of Child Psychiatry.* Norton, New York, 1963. pp. 60–71.

Anders, T. F., and Weinstein, P. "Sleep and Its Disorders in Infants and Children: A Review." In: *Annual Progress in Child Psychiatry and Child Development: 1973.* S. Chess and A. Thomas (eds.). Brunner/Mazel, New York, 1974. pp. 377–395.

Andronico, M. P., Fidler, J., Guerney, B., Jr., and Guerney, L. F. "The Combination of Didactic and Dynamic Elements in a Filial Therapy." *Int. J. Group Psychother.* 17:10–17, 1967.

Annell, A. L. "Lithium in the Treatment of Children and Adolescents." *Acta Psychiatr. Scand.* 207(Suppl.): 19–33, 1969.

Anthony, E. J. "Psychoneurotic Disorders." In: *Comprehensive Textbook of Psychiatry.* A. M. Freedman and H. I. Kaplan (eds.). Williams & Wilkins, Baltimore, 1967. pp. 1387–1406.

Anthony, E. J., and Scott, P. "Manic–Depressive Psychosis in Childhood." *J. Child Psychol. Psychiatry Allied Discip.* 1:53–72, 1960.

Axelrod, S. "Symposium, 1955: Progress in Orthopsychiatry. Allied Disciplines." *Am. J. Orthopsychiatry* 25:524–538, 1955.

Barhash, A. Z., *et al.* "Appraising the Contribution of the Mental Hygiene Clinic to Its Community. 3. Discussion." *Am. J. Orthopsychiatry* 21:94–104, 1951.

Bateson, G., Jackson, D. D., Haley, J., and Weakland, M. "Toward a Theory of Schizophrenia." *Behav. Sci.* 1:251–264, 1956.

Behrens, M. L., and Goldfarb, W. "A Study of Patterns of Interaction of Families of Schizophrenic Children in Residential Treatment." *Am. J. Orthopsychiatry* 28:300–312, 1958.

Bell, N. W., and Vogel, E. F. "The Emotionally Disturbed Child as the Family Scapegoat." In: *A Modern Introduction to the Family.* N. W. Bell and E. F. Vogel (eds.). Free Press, New York, 1968. pp. 412–427.

Bender, L. *Psychopathology of Children with Organic Brain Disorders.* Charles C. Thomas, Springfield, Illinois, 1956.

Bender, L. "Autism in Children with Mental Deficiency." *Am. J. Ment. Defic.* 64:81–86, 1959.

Bender, L., and Gureivitz, S. "Results of Psychotherapy with Young Schizophrenic Children." *Am. J. Orthopsychiatry* 25:162–170, 1955.

Benedek, T. "The Psychosomatic Implications of the Primary Unit: Mother–Child." *Am. J. Orthopsychiatry* 19:642–654, 1949.

Benedek, T. "The Family as a Psychologic Field." In: *Parenthood: Its Psychology and Psychopathology.* E. J. Anthony and T. Benedek (eds.). Little, Brown, Boston, 1970a. pp. 109–136.

Benedek, T. "The Psychobiology of Pregnancy." In: *Parenthood.* E. J. Anthony and T. Benedek (eds.). Little, Brown, Boston, 1970b. pp. 137–151.

Berkowitz, P. H. "Some Psychophysical Aspects of Mental Illness in Children." *Genet. Psychol. Monogr.* 63:103–148, 1961.

Berlin, I. N. "Consultation and Special Education." In: *Prevention and Treatment of Mental Retardation.* I. Philips (ed.). Basic Books, New York, 1966. pp. 279–293.

Berlin, I. N. "An Early-Warning System of Detecting Childhood Problems." *Med. Insight* 1:11–15, 1969.

Berlin, I. N. *Bibliography for Training in Child Psychiatry* (Official Publication of the American Academy of Child Psychiatry). Human Sciences Press, New York, 1976.

Berlin, I. N., and Szurek, S. A. (eds.). *Learning and Its Disorders.* Science and Behavior Books, Palo Alto, 1965.

Berlin, I. N., and Szurek, S. A. "Parental Blame: An Obstacle in Psychotherapeutic Work with Schizophrenic Children and Their Families." In: *Clinical Studies in Childhood Psychoses.* S. A. Szurek and I. N. Berlin (eds.). Brunner/Mazel, New York, 1973. pp. 115–126.

Berman, S. "Alienation: An Essential Process of the Psychology of Adolescence." *J. Am. Acad. Child Psychiatry* 9:233–250, 1970.

Bettelheim, B. "Childhood Schizophrenia. Symposium, 1955. 3. Schizophrenia as a Reaction to Extreme Situations." *Am. J. Orthopsychiatry* 26:507–518, 1956.

Bibring, G. L., Dwyer, T. F., Huntington, D. S., and Valenstein, A. F. "A Study of the Psychological Processes in Pregnancy and of the Earliest Mother–Child Relationship. II. Methodological Considerations." *Psychoanal. Study Child* 16:25–72, 1961.

Biller, H. B. "A Note on Father Absence and Masculine Development in Lower-Class Negro and White Boys. *Child Dev.* 39:1003–1006, 1968.

Birch, H. G. "Malnutrition, Learning, and Intelligence." In: *Annual Progress in Child Psychiatry and Child Development: 1973*. S. Chess and A. Thomas (eds.). Brunner/Mazel, New York, 1974. pp. 321–346.

Birch, H. G., and Gussow, J. D. *Disadvantaged Children: Health, Nutrition, and School Failure*. Grune & Stratton, New York, 1970.

Blatt, A. "Group Therapy with Parents of Severely Retarded Children: A Preliminary Report." *Group Psychother.* **10**:133–140, 1957.

Blos, P. "Intensive Psychotherapy in Relation to the Various Phases of the Adolescent Period." *Am. J. Orthopsychiatry* **32**:901–910, 1962.

Blos, P. "The Second Individuation Process of Adolescence." *Psychoanal. Study Child* **22**:162–186, 1967.

Book, J. A., Nichtern, S., and Gruenberg, E. "Cytogenetical Investigations in Childhood Schizophrenia." *Acta Psychiatr. Scand.* **39**:9–323, 1963.

Boszormenyi-Nagy, I., and Framo, J. L. *Intensive Family Therapy: Theoretical and Practical Aspects*. Harper & Row, New York, 1965.

Bowen, M. "The Use of Family Theory in Clinical Practice." *Compr. Psychiatry* **7**:345–374, 1966.

Bronfenbrenner, U. "Socialization and Social Class Through Time and Space." In: *Society for the Psychological Study of Social Issues: Readings in Social Psychology*. 3rd ed. Holt, Rinehart & Winston, New York, 1958. pp. 400–425.

Bronfenbrenner, U. "Toward a Theoretical Model for the Analysis of Parent–Child Relationships in a Social Context." In: *Parental Attitudes and Child Behavior*. J. C. Glidewell (ed.). Charles C. Thomas, Springfield, Illinois, 1961. pp. 90–109.

Call, J. D. "Prevention of Autism in a Young Infant in a Well-Child Conference." *J. Am. Acad. Child Psychiatry* **2**:451–459, 1963.

Caplan, G., Mason, E. A., and Kaplan, D. M. "Four Studies of Crisis in Parents of Prematures." *Community Ment. Health J.* **1**:149–161, 1965.

Cassell, J. "Social Class and Mental Disorders: An Analysis of the Limitations and Potentialities of Current Epidemiological Approaches." In: *Mental Health and the Lower Classes*. K. S. Miller and C. M. Grigg (eds.). Florida State University Press, Tallahassee, 1966. pp. 42–53.

Chafetz, M. E., Blane, H. T., and Hill, M. J. "Children of Alcoholics: Observations in a Child Guidance Clinic." *Q. J. Stud. Alcohol* **32**:687–698, 1971.

Chan, A., Chin, A., and Mueller, D. J., "An Integrated Approach to the Modification of Classroom Failure and Disruption: A Case Study." *J. School Psychol.* **8**:114–121, 1970.

Chase, A. *The Biological Imperatives: Health, Politics, and Human Survival*. Holt, Rinehart & Winston, New York, 1971.

Cheney, K. B. "Safeguarding Legal Rights in Providing Protective Services." *Children* **13**:87–92, 1966.

Chess, S. "Diagnosis and Treatment of the Hyperactive Child." *N.Y. State J. Med.* **60**:2379–2385, 1960.

Chess, S. "Neurological Dysfunction and Childhood Behavioral Pathology." *J. Autism Child. Schizophr.* **2**:299–311, 1972.

Chess, S., and Thomas, A. "Differences in Outcome with Early Intervention in Children with Behavior Disorders." In: *Life History Research in Psychopathology*. M. Roff, L. N. Robins, and M. Pollack (eds.). Vol. 2. University of Minnesota Press, Minneapolis, 1972. pp. 35–46.

Chess, S., Thomas, A., and Birch, H. G. "Behavior Problems Revisited: Findings of an Anterospective Study." *J. Am. Acad. Child Psychiatry* **6**:321–331, 1967.

Clausen, J. A. "Family Structure, Socialization, and Personality." *Rev. Child Dev. Res.* **2**:1–53, 1966.

Clement, P. W. "Please Mother, I'd Rather You Did It Yourself: Training Parents to Treat Their Own Children." *J. School Health* **41**:65–69, 1971.

Cohen, R. L., Charny, I. W., and Lembke, P. "Parental Expectations as a Force in Treatment: The Identification of Unconscious Parental Projections onto the Children's Psychiatric Hospital." *Arch. Gen. Psychiatry* **4**:471–478, 1961.

Cohen, R. L., Rose, J., and Henderson, P. B. *A Handbook of Developmental Interviewing*. Rev. ed. University of Pittsburgh, Department of Psychiatry, Division of Child Psychiatry Training Manual (available from authors), 1975.

Coppolillo, H. P. "A Technical Consideration in Child Analysis and Child Therapy." *J. Am. Acad. Child Psychiatry* **8**:411–435, 1969.

Cravioto, J. "Nutritional Deficiencies and Mental Performance in Childhood." In: *Environmental Influences: Proceedings of a Conference under the Auspices of Russell Sage Foundation and the Rockefeller University*. D. C. Glass (ed.). Rockefeller University Press, New York, 1968. pp. 3–51.

Curran, W. J. "The Revolution in American Criminal Law: Its Significance for Psychiatric Diagnosis and Treatment." *Am. J. Public Health* **58:**2209–2216, 1968.

Cytryn, L., and McKnew, D. H., Jr. "Proposed Classification of Childhood Depression." In: *Annual Progress in Child Psychiatry and Child Development: 1973*. S. Chess and A. Thomas (eds.). Brunner/Mazel, New York, 1974. pp. 419–432.

Davids, A., Ryan, R., and Salvatore, P. D. "Effectiveness of Residential Treatment for Psychotic and Other Disturbed Children." *Am. J. Orthopsychiatry* **38:**469–475, 1968.

DeHirsch, K. "A Review of Early Language Development." *Dev. Med. Child Neurol.* **12:**87–97, 1970.

Deutsch, C. P. "Social Class and Child Development." In: *Review of Child Development Research*. B. M. Caldwell and H. N. Ricciuti (eds.). Vol. 3. *Child Development and Social Policy*. University of Chicago Press, 1973. pp. 233–282.

Douglas, J. W., and Mulligan, D. G. "Emotional Adjustment and Educational Achievement: The Preliminary Results of a Longitudinal Study of a National Sample of Children." *Proc. R. Soc. Med.* **54:**885–891, 1961.

Dubin, R., and Dubin, E. R. "Children's Social Perceptions: A Review of Research." *Child Dev.* **36:**809–838, 1965.

Dubos, R. "Environmental Determinants of Human Life." In: *Environmental Influences: Proceedings of a Conference Under the Auspices of Russell Sage Foundation and the Rockefeller University*. D. C. Glass (ed.). Rockefeller University Press, New York, 1968. pp. 138–154.

Eisenberg, L. "Emotional Determinants of Mental Deficiency." *Arch. Neurol. Psychiatry* **80:**114–141, 1958*a*.

Eisenberg, L. "School Phobia: A Study in the Communication of Anxiety." *Am. J. Psychiatry* **114:**712–718, 1958*b*.

Eisenberg, L. "The Classification of the Psychotic Disorders in Childhood." In: *The Classification of Behavior Disorders*. L. D. Eron (ed.). Aldine, Chicago, 1966. pp. 87–114.

Eisenberg, L. "Child Psychiatry: The Past Quarter Century." *Am. J. Orthopsychiatry* **39:**389–401, 1969.

Ekstein, R., and Wallerstein, J. "Observations on the Psychotherapy of Borderline and Psychotic Children." *Psychoanal. Study Child* **11:**303–311, 1956.

Ekstein, R., and Wallerstein, J. "Choice of Interpretation in the Treatment of Borderline and Psychotic Children." *Bull. Menninger Clin.* **21:**199–207, 1957.

Ekstein, R., Wallerstein, J., and Mandelbaum, A. "Counter-Transference in the Residential Treatment of Children: Treatment Failure in a Child with Symbiotic Psychosis." *Psychoanal. Study Child* **14:**186–218, 1959.

Emmerich, W. "Personality Development and Concepts of Structure." *Child Dev.* **39:**671–690, 1968.

Engel, G. L. "Is Grief a Disease? A Challenge for Medical Research." *Psychosom. Med.* **23:**18–22, 1961.

Erikson, E. H. "The Problem of Ego Identity." *J. Am. Psychoanal. Assoc.* **4:**56–121, 1956.

Erikson, E. H. *Identity and the Life Cycle*. International Universities Press, New York, 1959. (*Psychological Issues* **1**, No. 1, 1959.)

Erikson, E. H. "The Theory of Infantile Sexuality." In: *Childhood and Society*. Norton, New York, 1963*a*. pp. 48–108.

Erikson, E. H. *Childhood and Society*. 2nd ed. Norton, New York, 1963*b*.

Escalona, S. K., and Heider, G. M. *Prediction and Outcome*. Basic Books, New York, 1959.

Ferber, A., Mendelsohn, M., and Napier, A. *The Book of Family Therapy*. Science House, New York, 1972.

Fish, B. "Longitudinal Observations of Biological Deviations in a Schizophrenic Infant." *Am. J. Psychiatry* **116:**25–31, 1959.

Fish, B. "Drug Therapy in Child Psychiatry: Pharmacological Aspects." *Compr. Psychiatry* **1:**212–227, 1960

Fish, B. "Drug Use in Psychiatric Disorders of Children." *Am. J. Psychiatry* **124**(No. 8 Supplement):31–36, 1968.

Fish, B. "Limitations of the New Nomenclature for Children's Disorders." *Int. J. Psychiatry* **7:**393–398, 1969.

Fish, B. "The 'One Child, One Drug' Myth of Stimulants in Hyperkinesis: Importance of Diagnostic Categories in Evaluating Treatment." *Arch. Gen. Psychiatry* **25**:193–203, 1971.

Fish, B., and Shapiro, T. "A Typology of Children's Psychiatric Disorders. I. Its Application to a Controlled Evaluation of Treatment." *J. Am. Acad. Child Psychiatry* **4**:32–52, 1965.

Fleck, S. "An Approach to Family Psychotherapy." *Compr. Psychiatry* **7**(5):307–320, October 1966.

Fleming, J. "Teaching the Basic Skills of Psychotherapy." *Arch. Gen. Psychiatry* **16**:416–426, 1967.

Foster, H. H. "Adoption and Child Custody: Best Interests of the Child?" *Buffalo Law Rev.* **22**:1–16, 1973.

Freeman, R. D. "Psychopharmacology and the Retarded Child." In: *Psychiatric Approaches to Mental Retardation.* F. J. Menolascino (ed.). Basic Books, New York, 1970. pp. 294–368.

Freud, A. *The Ego and the Mechanisms of Defense* (*Writings*, Vol. 2). International Universities Press, New York, 1946.

Freud, A. "The Assessment of Normality in Childhood." In: *Normality and Pathology in Childhood* (*Writings*, Vol. 6). Hogarth Press, London, 1966a. pp. 54–107.

Freud, A. *Normality and Pathology in Childhood* (*Writings*, Vol. 6). Hogarth Press, London, 1966b. pp. 149–164.

Freud, A. "The Symptomatology of Childhood: A Preliminary Attempt at Classification." *Psychoanal. Study Child* **25**:19–41, 1970.

Freud, A., and Dann, S. "An Experiment in Group Upbringing" (*Writings*, Vol. 4, pp. 163–229). *Psychoanal. Study Child* **6**:127–168, 1951.

Freud, S. (1905) "The Period of Sexual Latency in Childhood and Its Interruptions." In: *Standard Edition*, Vol. 7, pp. 176–179. Hogarth Press, London, 1953a.

Freud, S. (1905) "Three Essays on the Theory of Sexuality." In: *Standard Edition*, Vol. 7, pp. 135–243. Hogarth Press, London, 1953b.

Group for the Advancement of Psychiatry: Committee on Adolescence. "Normal Adolescence." GAP Report No. 68. Group for the Advancement of Psychiatry, New York, 1968.

Group for the Advancement of Psychiatry: Committee on Child Psychiatry. "Psychopathological Disorders in Childhood: Theoretical Considerations and a Proposed Classification." GAP Report No. 62. Group for the Advancement of Psychiatry, New York, 1966.

Group for the Advancement of Psychiatry: Committee on Child Psychiatry. "From Diagnosis to Treatment: An Approach to Treatment Planning for the Emotionally Disturbed Child." GAP Report No. 87. Group for the Advancement of Psychiatry, New York, 1973.

Group for the Advancement of Psychiatry: Committee on Public Education. "The Joys and Sorrows of Parenthood." GAP Report No. 84. Group for the Advancement of Psychiatry, New York, 1973.

Gesell, A. L., and Amatruda, C. S. *Developmental Diagnosis: Normal and Abnormal Child Development, Clinical Methods and Pediatric Applications.* 2nd ed. Hoeber, New York, 1947.

Gil, T. D. "The Legal Nature of Neglect." *Crime and Delinquency* **6**:1–16, 1960.

Ginott, H. G. "Group Therapy with Children." In: *Basic Approaches to Group Psychotherapy and Group Counseling.* G. M. Gazda (ed.). Charles C. Thomas, Springfield, Illinois, 1968. pp. 176–194.

Glaser, K. "Masked Depression in Children and Adolescents." *Am. J. Psychotherapy* **21**:565–574, 1967.

Goldfarb, W., and Forsen, M. M. *Annotated Bibliography of Childhood Schizophrenia and Related Disorders.* Basic Books, New York, 1956.

Goldstein, J., Freud, A., and Solnit, A. J. *Beyond the Best Interests of the Child.* Free Press, New York, 1970.

Graffagnino, P. N., Boelhouwer, C., and Reznikoff, M. "An Organic Factor in Patients of a Child Psychiatric Clinic: Data from the Early Interviews and the Electroencephalogram." *J. Am. Acad. Child Psychiatry* **7**:618–638, 1968.

Grant, Q. R. "Psychopharmacology in Childhood Emotional and Mental Disorders." *J. Pediatr.* **61**:626–637, 1962.

Green, M. "Care of the Child with a Long-Term, Life-Threatening Illness: Some Principles of Management." *Pediatrics* **39**: 441–445, 1967.

Greenbaum, H. "Marriage, Family and Parenthood." *Am. J. Psychiatry* **130**:1262–1265, 1973.

Gregory, I. "Genetic Factors in Schizophrenia." *Am. J. Psychiatry* **116**:961–972, 1960.

Gruenberg, E. M., and Leighton, A. H. "Epidemiology and Psychiatric Training." In: *Concepts of*

Community Psychiatry: A Framework for Training. S. E. Goldston (ed.). U.S. National Institute of Mental Health, Bethesda, Maryland, 1965. pp. 109–115.

Harris, D. B., and Roberts, J. *Intellectual Maturity of Children: Demographic and Socioeconomic Factors, United States.* (Vital and Health Statistics, Ser. 11, No. 116.) [DHEW Publ. No. (HSM) 72-1059.] U.S. Health Services and Mental Health Administration, Rockville, Maryland, 1972.

Harrison, S. I. "Reared in the Wrong Sex." *J. Am. Acad. Child Psychiatry* 9:44–102, 1970.

Heeley, A. F., and Roberts, G. E. "Tryptophan Metabolism in Psychotic Children." *Dev. Med. Child Neurol.* 7:46–49, 1965.

Henderson, P. B. "Basic Essentials in the Training and Education of the Child Psychiatrist." Final draft in preparation, American Academy of Child Psychiatry, Committee on Training, 1977.

Henry, J. "The Culture of Interpersonal Relations in a Therapeutic Institution for Emotionally Disturbed Children." *Am. J. Orthopsychiatry* 27:725–734, 1957.

Hersov, L. A. "Refusal to Go to School." *J. Child Psychol. Psychiatry Allied Discip.* 1:137–145, 1960.

Hess, E. H. "Imprinting in Birds." *Science* 146:1128–1139, 1964.

Hess, R. D. "Social Class and Ethnic Influences upon Socialization." In: *Manual of Child Psychology.* L. Carmichael (ed.). Vol. 2. 3rd ed. Wiley, New York, 1970. pp. 457–557.

Hess, R. D., and Shipman, V. C. "Early Experience and the Socialization of Cognitive Modes in Children." *Child Dev.* 36:869–886, 1965.

Hetznecker, W., and Forman, M. A. "Community Child Psychiatry: Evolution and Direction." *Am. J. Orthopsychiatry* 41: 350–370, 1971.

Hingtgen, J. N., and Bryson, C. Q. "Recent Developments in the Study of Early Childhood Psychoses: Infantile Autism, Childhood Schizophrenia, and Related Disorders." In: *Annual Progress in Child Psychiatry and Child Development: 1973.* S. Chess and A. Thomas (eds.). Brunner/ Mazel, New York, 1974. pp. 503–575.

Howell, M. C., Emmons, E. B., and Frank, D. A. "Reminiscences of Runaway Adolescents." *Am. J. Orthopsychiatry* 43:840–853, 1973.

Jackson, D. D. "Family Interaction, Family Homeostasis and Some Implications for Conjoint Family Psychotherapy." *Science Psychoanal.* 2:122–141, 1959.

Jackson, D. D. "A Critique of the Literature on the Genetics of Schizophrenia." In: *The Etiology of Schizophrenia.* Basic Books, New York, 1960. pp. 37–87.

Jakab, I. "Psychotherapy of the Mentally Retarded Child." In: *Diminished People.* N. R. Bernstein (ed.). Little, Brown, Boston, 1970. pp. 223–261.

Jensen, A. A. "A Theory of Primary and Secondary Familial Mental Retardation." *Int. Rev. Res. Ment. Retard.* 4:33–106, 1970.

Jessner, L., Weigert, E., and Foy, J. L. "The Development of Parental Attitudes During Pregnancy." In: *Parenthood.* E. J. Anthony and T. Benedek (eds.). Little, Brown, Boston, 1970. pp. 209–244.

Johnson, A. M., and Robinson, D. B. "The Sexual Deviant (Sexual Psychopath)—Causes, Treatment, and Prevention." *J. Am. Med. Assoc.* 164:1559–1565, 1957.

Johnson, A. M., Falstein, E. I., Szurek, S. A., and Svendsen, M. "School Phobia." *Am. J. Orthopsychiatry* 11:702–711, 1941.

Joint Commission on Mental Health of Children. *Crisis in Child Mental Health: Challenge for the 1970's.* Harper & Row, New York, 1970.

Joint Commission on Mental Health of Children. *Mental Health: From Infancy through Adolescence; Reports of Task Forces I, II, and III and the Committee on Education and Religion.* Harper & Row, New York, 1973.

Judd, L. L., and Mandell, A. J. "Chromosome Studies in Early Infantile Autism." *Arch. Gen. Psychiatry* 18:450–457, 1968.

Kalish, R. A. "Death and Bereavement: A Bibliography." *J. Hum. Relations* 13:118–141, 1965.

Kamii, C. K., and Radin, N. L. "Class Differences in the Socialization Practices of Negro Mothers." *J. Marriage Family* 29:302–310, 1967.

Kanner, L. "Autistic Disturbances of Affective Contact." *Nerv. Child* 2:217–250, 1943.

Kanner, L. "Early Infantile Autism." *J. Pediatr.* 25:211–217, 1944.

Karpman, B., *et al.* "A Differential Study of Psychopathic Behavior in Infants and Children." Round Table, 1951. *Am. J. Orthopsychiatry* 22:223–267, 1952.

Kempf, J. P. "Communicating with the Psychotic Child." *Int. Psychiatry Clin.* 1(1):53–72, 1964.

Kessler, J. W. "Nosology in Child Psychopathology." In: *Perspectives in Child Psychopathology.* H. E. Rie (ed.). Aldine-Atherton, Chicago, 1971. pp. 85–129.

Kleinfield, A. J. "The Balance of Power among Infants, Their Parents, and the State." *Family Law Q.* 5:63–107, 1971.

Klerman, G. L. "The Teaching of Psychopharmacology in the Psychiatric Residency." *Compr. Psychiatry* 6:255–264, 1965.

Konopka, G. "The Role of Residential Treatment for Children. Symposium, 1954. 4. The Role of the Group in Residential Treatment." *Am. J. Orthopsychiatry* 25:679–684, 1955.

Koppitz, E. M. "Psychotherapy and Children's Drawings." In: *Psychological Evaluation of Children's Figure Drawings*. Grune & Stratton, New York, 1968. pp. 245–257.

Koupernik, C. "The Roots of Hypochondriasis in the Child." In: *The Child in His Family*. Vol. 2. *The Impact of Disease and Death*. E. J. Anthony and C. Koupernik (eds.). Wiley, New York, pp. 85–95. (*International Yearbook for Child Psychiatry and Allied Disciplines*, Vol. 2.)

Kreitler, H., and Kreitler, S. "Children's Concepts of Sexuality and Birth." *Child Dev.* 37:363–378, 1966.

Kris, M. "The Use of Prediction in a Longitudinal Study." *Psychoanal. Study Child* 12:175–189, 1957.

Kysar, J. E. "Reactions of Professionals to Disturbed Children and Their Parents." *Arch. Gen. Psychiatry* 19:562–570, 1968.

Langner, T. S., *et al.* "Children of the City: Affluence, Poverty, and Mental Health." In: *Psychological Factors in Poverty*. V. L. Allen (ed.). Markham, Chicago, 1970. pp. 185–209.

LaVietes, R. L., Hulse, W. C., and Blau, A. "A Psychiatric Day Treatment Center and School for Young Children and Their Parents." *Am. J. Orthopsychiatry* 30:468–482, 1960.

Levine, M., and Levine, A. *A Social History of Helping Services: Clinic, Court, School and Community*. Appleton-Century-Crofts, New York, 1970.

LeVine, R. A. "Cross-Cultural Study in Child Psychology. In: *Manual of Child Psychology*. L. Carmichael (ed.). Vol. 2. 3rd ed. Wiley, New York, 1970. pp. 559–612.

Levy, D. M. "Beginnings of the Child Guidance Movement." *Am. J. Orthopsychiatry* 38:799–804, 1968.

Lewis, M., and Sarrel, P. M., "Some Psychological Aspects of Seduction, Incest, and Rape in Childhood." *J. Am. Acad. Child Psychiatry* 8:606–619, 1969.

Lewis, O. *Five Families*. Basic Books, New York, 1959.

Lidz, T. F. "Schizophrenia and the Family." *Psychiatry* 21:21–27, 1958.

Lidz, T. F. "The Marital Relationship, Family Structure and Personality Development." In: *Proceedings of the Third World Congress of Psychiatry: 1961*. Vol. 3. University of Toronto Press, Montreal, 1961–1963. pp. 117–120.

Lidz, T. F., Cornelison, A. R., Fleck, S., and Terry, D. "The Intrafamilial Environment of the Schizophrenic Patient. I. The Father." *Psychiatry* 20:329–342, 1957.

Lindemann, E. "Symptomatology and Management of Acute Grief." *Am. J. Psychiatry* 101:141–148, 1944.

Loesch, J. G., and Greenberg, N. H. "Some Specific Areas of Conflicts Observed during Pregnancy: A Comparative Study of Married and Unmarried Pregnant Women." *Am. J. Orthopsychiatry* 32:624–636, 1962.

Lowrey, L. G. "The Contribution of Orthopsychiatry to Psychiatry: Brief Historical Note." *Am. J. Orthopsychiatry* 25:475–478, 1955.

Lytton, H. "Observation Studies of Parent–Child Interaction: A Methodological Review." *Child Dev.* 42:651–684, 1971.

MacGregor, R., *et al. Multiple Impact Therapy with Families*. McGraw-Hill, New York, 1964.

Mahler, M. S. "On Childhood Psychosis and Schizophrenia: Autistic and Symbiotic Infantile Psychoses." *Psychoanal. Study Child* 7:286–305, 1952.

Mahler, M. S. "On Human Symbiosis and the Vicissitudes of Individuation." *J. Am. Psychoanal. Assoc.* 15:740–763, 1967.

Malone, C. A. "Child Psychiatric Services for Low Socioeconomic Families." *J. Am. Acad. Child Psychiatry* 6:332–345, 1967.

Mattsson, A. "The Male Therapist and the Female Adolescent Patient." *J. Am. Acad. Child Psychiatry* 9:707–721, 1970.

Mattsson, A., Seese, L. R., and Hawkins, J. W. "Suicidal Behavior as a Child Psychiatric Emergency: Clinical Characteristics and Follow-Up Results." *Arch. Gen. Psychiatry* 20:100–109, 1969.

Matza, D. *Becoming Deviant*. Prentice-Hall, Englewood Cliffs, New Jersey, 1969.

McDermott, J. F., McGuire, C., and Berner, E. F. *Roles and Functions of Child Psychiatrists*. The Committee on Certification in Child Psychiatry of the American Board of Psychiatry and Neurology, 1976.

McNickle, D. "The Sociocultural Setting of Indian Life." *Am. J. Psychiatry* **125**:219-223, 1968.

Mead, M. *From the South Seas: Studies of Adolescence and Sex in Primitive Societies.* Morrow, New York, 1939.

Meeks, J. E. *The Fragile Alliance: An Orientation to the Outpatient Psychotherapy of the Adolescent.* Williams & Wilkins, Baltimore, 1971.

Menolascino, F. J. "Psychiatry's Past, Current and Future Role in Mental Retardation." In: *Psychiatric Approaches to Mental Retardation.* Basic Books, New York, 1970. pp. 709-744.

Mercer, J. R. "A Policy Statement on Assessment Procedures and the Rights of Children." *Harv. Educational Rev.* **44**:125-141, 1974.

Miller, E. "The Problem of Classification in Child Psychiatry (Some Epidemiological Considerations). In: *Foundations of Child Psychiatry.* Pergamon, Oxford, 1968. pp. 251-269.

Miller, L. "Child Rearing in the Kibbutz." In: *Modern Perspectives in International Child Psychiatry (Modern Perspectives in Psychiatry,* Vol. 3). J. G. Howells (ed.). Oliver & Boyd, Edinburgh, 1969. pp. 321-346.

Millichap, J. G. "Drugs in Management of Hyperkinetic and Perceptually Handicapped Children." *J. Am. Med. Assoc.* **206**:1527-1530, 1968.

Minuchin, P. P., Bier, B., *et al. The Psychological Impact of School Experience.* Basic Books, New York, 1969.

Minuchin, S. "Conflict-Resolution Family Therapy." *Psychiatry* **28**: 278-286, 1965.

Minuchin, S. *Families and Family Therapy: A Structural Approach.* Harvard Press, Cambridge, 1974.

Minuchin, S., and Montalvo, B. "Techniques for Working with Disorganized Low Socioeconomic Families." *Am. J. Orthopsychiatry* **37**:880-887, 1967.

Monroe, R. R., Klee, G. D., and Brody, E. B. "Psychiatric Epidemiology and Mental Health Planning." *Psychiatr. Res. Rep.* **22**, 1967.

Nagera, H. "On Arrest in Development, Fixation, and Regression." *Psychoanal. Study Child* **19**:222-239, 1964.

Nagera, H. "Children's Reactions to the Death of Important Objects: A Developmental Approach." *Psychoanal. Study Child* **25**:360-400, 1970.

Naughton, F. X. "Foster Home Placement as an Adjunct to Residential Treatment." *Soc. Casework* **38**:288-295, 1957.

Nolfi, M. W. "Families in Grief: The Question of Casework Intervention." *Soc. Work* **12**(4):40-46, 1967.

Noshpitz, J. D. "Certain Cultural and Familial Factors Contributing to Adolescent Alienation." *J. Am. Acad. Child Psychiatry* **9**:216-223, 1970.

Offer, D., and Offer, J. "Four Issues in the Developmental Psychology of Adolescents." In: *Modern Perspectives in Adolescent Psychiatry (Modern Perspectives in Psychiatry,* Vol. 4). J. G. Howells (ed.). Oliver & Bond, Edinburgh, 1971. pp. 28-44.

Offord, D. R., and Aponte, J. F. "Distortion of Disability and Effect on Family Life." *J. Am. Acad. Child Psychiatry* **6**:499-511, 1967.

Paredes, A., Hood, W. R., and Gregory, D. "Microecology of Alcoholism: Implications for the Development of the Adolescent." In: *Current Issues in Adolescent Psychiatry.* J. C. Schoolar (ed.). Brunner/Mazel, New York, 1973. pp. 158-178.

Pearson, G. H. "A Survey of Learning Difficulties in Children." *Psychoanal. Study Child* **7**:322-386, 1952.

Penick, S. B., Filion, R., Fox, S., and Stunkard, A. J. *Psychosom. Med.* **33**:49-55, 1971.

Philips, I. "Problems of Training the Professional in the Field of Mental Retardation: A Review of a Training Program." *J. Am. Acad. Child Psychiatry* **5**:693-705, 1966.

Piaget, J. "Piaget's Theory." In: *Manual of Child Psychology.* L. Carmichael (ed.). Vol. 1. 3rd ed. Wiley, New York, 1970. pp. 703-732.

Proposed Revised Uniform Marriage and Divorce Act. *Family Law Q.* **7**:135-167, 1973.

Prugh, D. G., Staub, E. M., Sands, H. H., Kirschbaum, R. M., and Lenihan, E. A. "A Study of the Emotional Reactions of Children and Families to Hospitalization and Illness." *Am. J. Orthopsychiatry* **23**:70-106, 1953.

Rabinovitch, R. D. "An Evaluation of Present Trends in Psychotherapy with Children." In: *Child Psychotherapy.* M. R. Haworth (ed.). Basic Books, New York, 1964. pp. 39-45.

Rae-Grant, Q. A. F., and Marcuse, D. J. "The Hazards of Teamwork." *Am. J. Orthopsychiatry* **38**:4-8, 1968.

Rank, B., and Kaplan, S. "A Case of Pseudoschizophrenia in a Child." Workshop, 1950. *Am. J. Ortho-psychiatry* **21**:155–181, 1951.

Rank, B., Putnam, M. C., and Rochlin, G. "The Significance of the 'Emotional Climate' in Early Feeding Difficulties." *Psychosom. Med.* **10**:279–283, 1948.

Redl, F. "The Concept of a 'Therapeutic Milieu.'" *Am. J. Orthopsychiatry* **29**:721–736, 1959.

Redl, F., and Wineman, D. *Children Who Hate.* Free Press, Glencoe, Illinois, 1951.

Reinhart, J. U. "The Doctor's Dilemma: Whether or Not to Recommend Continuous Renal Dialysis or Renal Homo-transplantation for the Child with End-Stage Renal Disease." *J. Pediatr.* **77**:505–506, 1970.

Rexford, E. N. "Children, Child Psychiatry, and Our Brave New World." *Arch. Gen. Psychiatry* **20**:25–37, 1969.

Rexford, E. N. Foreword to *Bibliography of Training in Child Psychiatry*, AACP Official Publication. Human Sciences Press, New York, 1976. pp. 1–3.

Rie, H. E. "Depression in Childhood: A Survey of Some Pertinent Contributions." *J. Am. Acad. Child Psychiatry* **5**:653–685, 1966.

Riskin, J., and Faunce, E. E. "An Evaluative Review of Family Interaction Research." *Fam. Process* **11**:365–455, 1972.

Rosenheim, M. D. "The Child and the Law." In: *Review of Child Development Research.* B. M. Caldwell and H. N. Ricciuti (eds.). Vol. 3. *Child Development and Social Policy.* University of Chicago Press, 1973. pp. 509–555.

Rubenstein, B. O., Falick, M. L., Levitt, M., and Ekstein, R. "Learning Problems. 2. Learning Impotence: A Suggested Diagnostic Category." *Am. J. Orthopsychiatry* **29**:315–323, 1959.

Rutter, M. "Normal Psychosexual Development." *J. Child Psychol. Psychiatry Allied Discip.* **11**:259–283, 1971.

Rutter, M. "Childhood Schizophrenia Reconsidered." *J. Autism Child. Schizophr.* **2**:315–337, 1972.

Rutter, M., *et al.* "A Tri-Axial Classification of Mental Disorders in Childhood: An International Study." *J. Child Psychol. Psychiatry Allied Discip.* **10**:41–61, 1969.

Sankar, S. D., Cates, N., Broer, H. H., and Sankar, D. B. "Biochemical Parameters of Childhood Schizophrenia (Autism) and Growth." *Recent Adv. Biol. Psychiatry* **5**:76–83, 1961.

Schain, R. J., and Freedman, D. X. "Studies on 5-Hydroxyindole Metabolism in Autistic and Other Mentally Retarded Children." *J. Pediatr.* **58**:315–320, 1961.

Scheibel, M. E., and Scheibel, A. B. "Some Neural Substrates of Postnatal Development." In: *Review of Child Development Research.* M. L. Hoffman and L. W. Hoffman (eds.). Vol. 1. Russell Sage Foundation, New York, 1964. pp. 481–519.

Schell, R. E., and Adams, W. P. "Training Parents of a Young Child with Profound Behavior Deficits to Be Teacher-Therapists." *J. Special Education* **2**:439–454, 1968.

Schofield, M. "Normal Sexuality in Adolescence." In: *Modern Perspectives in Adolescent Psychiatry* (*Modern Perspectives in Psychiatry*, Vol. 4). J. G. Howells (ed.). Oliver & Boyd, Edinburgh, 1971. pp. 45–65.

Schowalter, J. E., and Solnit, A. J. "Child Psychiatry Consultation in a General Hospital Emergency Room." *J. Am. Acad. Child Psychiatry* **5**:534–551, 1966.

Schuman, L. M. *Research Methodology and Potential in Community Health and Preventitive Medicine* [*Ann. N.Y. Acad. Sci.* **107**(Art. 2):471–808, 1962]. New York Academy of Sciences, New York, 1968.

Schur, M. "Comments on the Metapsychology of Somatization." *Psychoanal. Study Child* **10**:119–164, 1955.

Shapiro, T., Fish, B., and Ginsberg, G. L. "The Speech of a Schizophrenic Child from Two to Six." *Am. J. Psychiatry* **128**:1408–1413, 1972.

Shrand, H. "Behavior Changes in Sick Children Nursed at Home." *Pediatrics* **36**:604–607, 1965.

Solnit, A. J. "Hospitalization: An Aid to Physical and Psychological Health in Childhood." *Am. J. Dis. Child.* **99**:155–163, 1960.

Sperling, M. "Etiology and Treatment of Sleep Disturbances in Children." *Psychoanal. Q.* **24**:358–368, 1955.

Sperling, M. "Pavor Nocturnus." *J. Am. Psychiatr. Assoc.* **6**:79–94, 1958.

Spitz, R. A., and Wolf, K. M. "Anaclitic Depression. An Inquiry into the Genesis of Psychiatric Conditions in Early Childhood, II." *Psychoanal. Study Child* **2**:313–342, 1946.

Stennett, R. G. "Emotional Handicap in the Elementary Years: Phase or Disease?" *Am. J. Orthopsychiatry* **36**:444–449, 1966.

Straus, R. "Some Early Research on Drinking and Problem Drinking." *Psychiatr. Ann.* 3(10):13–14, 1973.

Szasz, T. S. "The Problem of Psychiatric Nosology." *Am. J. Psychiatry* **114**:405–413, 1957.

Sze, W. C. "Social Variables and Their Effect on Psychiatric Emergency Situations among Children." *Ment. Hyg.* **55**:437–443, 1971.

Szurek, S. A. "Comments on the Psychopathology of Children with Somatic Illness." *Am. J. Psychiatry* **107**:844–849, 1951.

Szurek, S. A. "Childhood Schizophrenia. Symposium, 1955. 4. Psychotic Episodes and Psychotic Maldevelopment." *Am. J. Orthopsychiatry* **26**:519–543, 1956.

Szurek, S. A., and Berlin, I. N. "Elements of Psychotherapeutics with the Schizophrenic Child and His Parents." *Psychiatry* **19**:1–9, 1956.

Szurek, S. A., and Philips, I. "Clinical Work and Clinical Research as Scientific Inquiry: Five Conceptual Barriers to Clinical Science." In: *Clinical Studies in Childhood Psychoses.* Brunner/Mazel, New York, 1973. pp. 278–302.

Tarjan, G. "Prevention, a Program Goal in Mental Deficiency." *Am. J. Ment. Defic.* **64**:4–11, 1959.

Thomas, A., and Chess, S. *Temperament and Development.* Brunner/Mazel, New York, 1977.

Thomas, A., Birch, H. G., Chess, S., and Robbins, L. C. "Individuality in Responses of Children to Similar Environmental Situations." *Am. J. Psychiatry* **117**:798–803, 1961.

Tseng, W.-S., Arensdorf, A. M., McDermott, J. F., *et al.* "Family Diagnosis and Classification." *J. Am. Acad. Child Psychiatry* **15**(1):15–35, 1976.

Valente, M., and Tarjan, G. "Etiologic Factors in Mental Retardation." *Psychiatr. Ann.* **4**(2):22–37, 1974.

Vandersall, T. A., and Weiner, J. M. "Children Who Set Fires." *Arch. Gen. Psychiatry* **22**:63–71, 1970.

Vernon, M. D. "The Development of Perception." In: *Modern Perspectives in Child Psychiatry* (*Modern Perspectives in Psychiatry*, Vol. 1). J. G. Howells (ed.). Oliver & Boyd, London, 1965.

Vogel, E. F. "The Marital Relationship of Parents of Emotionally Disturbed Children: Polarization and Isolation." *Psychiatry* **23**:1–12, 1960.

Walters, R. H., and Parke, R. D. "The Role of the Distance Receptors in the Development of Social Responsiveness." In: *Advances in Child Development and Behavior.* L. P. Lipsitt and C. C. Spiker (eds.). Vol. 2. Academic Press, New York, 1963. pp. 59–96.

Weiner, J. M. *Psychopharmacology in Childhood and Adolescence.* Basic Books, New York, 1977.

Weinrott, M. R. "A Training Program in Behavior Modification for Siblings of the Retarded." *Am. J. Orthopsychiatry* **44**:362–375, 1974.

Wender, P. H. *Minimal Brain Dysfunction in Children.* Wiley-Interscience, New York, 1971.

Werry, J. S., Weiss, G., and Douglas, V. "Studies on the Hyperactive Child. I: Some Preliminary Findings." *Can. Psychiatr. Assoc. J.* **9**:120–130, 1964.

Westman, J. C., and Cline, D. W. "Divorce Is a Family Affair." *Fam. Law Q.* **5**:1–10, 1971.

White, J. H., Nornsby, L. G., and Gordon, R. "Treating Infantile Autism with Parent Therapists." *Int. J. Child Psychother.* 1(3):83–95, 1972.

Williams, J. M. "Children Who Break Down in Foster Homes: A Psychological Study of Patterns of Personality Growth in Grossly Deprived Children." *J. Child Psychol. Psychiatry Allied Discip.* **2**:5–20, 1961.

Winnicott, D. W. "Growth and Development in Immaturity." In: *The Family and Individual Development.* Tavistock, London, 1965. pp. 21–29.

Witmer, H. L. *Psychiatric Clinics for Children.* Commonwealth Fund, New York, 1940.

Wolf, M. G. "Effects of Emotional Disturbance in Childhood on Intelligence." *Am. J. Orthopsychiatry* **35**:906–908, 1965.

Wolfensberger, W. "The Origin and Nature of Our Institutional Models." In: *Changing Patterns in Residential Services for the Mentally Retarded.* R. B. Kugel and W. Wolfensberger (eds.). President's Committee on Mental Retardation, Washington, D.C., 1969. pp. 59–171.

Wolff, P. H. "'Critical Periods' in Human Cognitive Development." *Hosp. Pract.* **5**(11):77–87, 1970.

Woltmann, A. G. "Concepts of Play Therapy Techniques." In: *Child Psychotherapy.* M. R. Haworth (ed.). Basic Books, New York, 1964. pp. 20–32.

Appendix A

Professional Associations

Residency training directors are frequently asked what professional associations a resident should join. Most often, the national organization plus one subspecialty organization are suggested, depending on the resident's areas of interest. If the addresses for such organizations are not available in one's education office, they can be easily obtained from a librarian, who will refer to such directories as the following:

A Directory of World Psychiatry
>   John Gunne (advisor to Hoffman LaRoche Ltd.) for the World Psychiatric Association, Switzerland, 1971. (350 pages)
>   Obtained through: The Maudsley Hospital, Denmark Hill, London, S.E. 5, England.

For every country in the world, this directory presents a brief description of the practice of psychiatry in that country, and a list and sometimes a description of the psychiatric hospitals, university departments, opportunities for foreign students, and types of research. In addition, it describes the general administration and organization of psychiatry, the national society, and the psychiatric journals. For many of the journals, the address and price are listed.

Encyclopedia of American Psychology and Psychiatry
>   Barry T. Klein, Todd Publications, Rye, New York, 1975. (459 pages)

This text lists various associations, research centers, periodicals, special libraries, foundations—grants and awards, audiovisual aids, psychiatric hospitals, mental health centers, psychology graduate schools, and psychiatric training programs. There is also a full subject-category index that lists, for each general subject area, all the associations, research centers, periodicals, special libraries, and audiovisual aids that relate to it.

Encyclopedia of Associations
>   Fisk, M., Wilson, M., Albright, J., National Organizations of the U.S., Vol. 1, Gale Research Co., Detroit, Michigan, 10th ed. 1976.

This text lists more than 60 psychiatric associations. For each association, it gives a brief description, address, phone number, founding date, and the number of members and staff and regional groups plus the names of its various councils and publications.

A few of the major organizations in the United States, Canada, Great Britain, and Australia are listed below with their present addresses. It is a short list and is meant only to provide an overview. Many major bodies in the English-speaking world that are omitted can easily be found in the texts listed above.

National Associations

The American Psychiatric Association
1700 Eighteenth Street, N.W.
Washington, D.C. 20009

The Royal Medico-Psychological
  Association
Chandos House
Queen Anne Street
London, W.1., England

The Australian and New Zealand College of Psychiatrists
Maudsley House
107 Rathdowne Street
Carleton, Victoria, Australia

The Canadian Psychiatric Associa-
  tion/Association des Psychiatres du
  Canada
Suite 103
225 Lisgar Street
Ottawa, K2P 0C6, Canada

Other Associations

The American Academy of Child Psychiatry
1800 R Street, Suite 904
Washington, D.C. 20009

C.O.P.E. (Co-ordinators of Psychiatric Education in Canada)
    The address of the General Secre-
tary can be obtained through the Canadian Psychiatric Association.

AADPRT (American Association of
  Directors of Psychiatric Residency
  Training)
Executive Office
The Institute of Living
200 Retreat Avenue
Hartford, Connecticut 06106

Specialist Examination Boards *
    Essentials of approved residency programs and requirements for sitting the specialist examinations can be obtained from:

---

*See Appendix C for official board and college information directly pertaining to required clinical and academic experiences. Paragraphs concerning requirements for physical and manpower program resources have not been quoted, but may be obtained from the appropriate source listed above.

Secretary, Liaison Committee on Graduate Education
American Medical Association
535 North Dearborn Street
Chicago, Illinois

Chief Co-Ordinating Secretary in Charge of Examinations
The Australian and New Zealand College of Psychiatrists
Private Bag 8, Post Office Parkville
Victoria 3052, Australia

Dean
Royal College of Psychiatrists
17 Belgrave Square
London, England SW1X 8PG

Director of Training and Evaluation
Royal College of Physicians and Surgeons of Canada
74 Stanley Avenue
Ottawa, Ontario, Canada K1P 1P4

Directories
  Association
  The Biographical Directory of the American Psychiatric Association
  Published for the American Psychiatric Association by R. R. Bowker Co., New York. 1977.
  Obtainable through the A.P.A.

  The Membership Directory of the American Psychiatric Association 1975
  American Psychiatric Association Publications Services Division
  1700 18th Street N.W.
  Washington, D.C. 20009

Other
The Directory of Clinical Fellowships in Medicine
   This directory can be obtained from Graduate Publications, Post Office Box 647, Glendale, California 91209.
   The directory lists over 3000 clinical fellowship programs in medicine for the United States and Canada. All medical subspecialty programs, including psychiatry, are listed. A fellowship is considered to be any type of postresidency training.

Appendix B

A Guide to the Psychiatric Literature

The literature in psychiatry is enormous. Residents may realistically feel overwhelmed. Although one's program director is the best source of advice concerning appropriate reading during different periods of training, this appendix provides an overview of some of the available basic literature.

Four textbooks are listed below mainly because of their proved popularity among residents, and one very short text is noted for those residents who would like to read a small book early in training to give them an overview of the field.

General Texts

Freedman, A. M., Kaplan, H. T., and Sadock, B. J. (eds.), *Comprehensive Textbook of Psychiatry II*, Williams & Wilkins Co., Baltimore, 1975.
Arieti, S. (ed.), *The American Handbook of Psychiatry*, 2nd ed., Basic Books Inc., New York, New York, 1974.
Slater, E., and Roth, M., *Clinical Psychiatry*, 3rd ed., Bailliere, Tindall and Cassell, Ltd., London, 1969.
Simons, R. C., and Pardes, H., *Understanding Human Behavior in Health and Illness*, Williams & Wilkins Co., Baltimore, 1977.
Merskey, H., and Tonge, W. L., *Psychiatric Illness*, 2nd ed., Bailliere, Tindall and Cassell Ltd., London, 1974.

There are, however, many other texts that deal with the entire field or with specific subtopic areas in it. A resident should ask the director of training and the librarian about which text will provide the clearest, most up-to-date perspective on the particular area being studied at any given time.

Reference Lists

In addition to textbooks, reference lists for more in-depth review of particular subject areas have been compiled by several organizations. These lists are updated every few years. Reference lists tend in all countries, however, to have a parochial slant—in Britain, from largely British literature; in North America, from North American journals. One can therefore find fault with any listing of references. For this reason, the editorial board recommends several sources for references.

Adult

British and Some European Literature

Kendell, R. E., and Smith, A. C. (eds.), The Royal College of Psychiatrists, Clinical Tutors Subcommittee, *Reading List in Psychiatry*, 4th ed., Headley Brothers' Ltd., Ashford, Kent, TN24 8HH, England, 40 pence.
   References noted in this list have been compiled in the following form:
Contemporary Psychiatry (ed. T. Silverstone and R. Barraclough), British Journal of Psychiatry Special Publication No. 9 (1975), H. Headley Brothers Ltd., Ashford, Kent, Tn24 8HH ($15.00).
A Compilation of Papers for the Use of Postgraduate Students of Psychiatry, 2nd ed. (ed. Barraclough, B., Heine, B., and Smith, A.), authorized by the Clinical Tutors Subcommittee of the Royal College of Psychiatrists, Great Britain. Available through Wyeth Ltd., Toronto, Ontario, Canada.

American Literature

Reading lists after each chapter in:
Freedman, A. M., Kaplan, H. T., and Sadock, B. J. (eds.), *Comprehensive Textbook of Psychiatry II*, Williams & Wilkins Co., Baltimore, 1975.
Arieti, S. (ed.), *The American Handbook of Psychiatry*, 2nd ed., Basic Books, Inc., New York, 1974.

Children

Berlin, I. N., *Bibliography of Child Psychiatry with Selected List of Films*, official publication of the American Academy of Child Psychiatry, Human Sciences Press, New York, 1976.
References listed after each chapter in:
Steinhauer, P. D., and Rae-Grant, Q. (eds.), *Psychological Problems of the Child and His Family*, MacMillan of Canada, Toronto, 1977 ($12.95).

   In addition to recommending the publications listed above, we have included as Appendix D a short list of references for each section of Chapter 1. This list is meant only as a guide to reading and *as a supplement* to the lists referred to above. It is *not* exhaustive. Indeed, the references listed are *not* meant to represent the most important papers for each topic, but are rather a list of a small number of publications that some program directors have found useful as an introduction for their residents to a topic area. The "major" references are intended only to give a basic introductory overview of the section referred to, while the "other" references are intended to give an introduction to the literature on specific subtopic areas within a given section. This short list is therefore only a supplementary guide and should be modified in accordance with the resident's teaching program and/or the reference list of the journal club at his or her teaching center.

Journals

Texts and reference lists serve as a baseline. To keep up to date, however, current journals must be read. The following list represents frequently used journals. Again, it must be emphasized that one should consult both with one's director of education and the librarian and carefully assess personal educational needs and requirements before selecting a small list of journals for regular perusal. Note that both prices and addresses change from time to time.

General Psychiatry

American Journal of Psychiatry, American Psychiatric Association, 1700 Eighteenth Street N.W., Washington, D.C. 20009 (approx. $19.00).

Archives of General Psychiatry, American Medical Association, 535 North Dearborn Street, Chicago, Illinois 60610 (approx. $28.00).

Australian & New Zealand Journal of Psychiatry, Ramsay Ware Stockland Ltd., 552–556 Victoria Street, North Melbourne, Victoria 3051 (approx. $20.00).

British Journal of Psychiatry, Royal College of Psychiatrists, Headley Brothers Ltd., Ashford, Kent 7N24 8HH (approx. $100.00).

Canadian Psychiatric Associatoin Journal, W. G. Triffin, C.P.A.J., 2 Tremont Crescent, Don Mills, Ontario M3B 2S1 (approx. $20.00).

Comprehensive Psychiatry, Grune & Stratton, Inc., 111 Fifth Avenue, New York, New York 10003 (approx. $36.00).

Diseases of the Nervous System, Physicians Postgraduate Press, P.O. Box 38293, Memphis, Tennessee 38138 (approx. $33.00).

Hospital & Community Psychiatry, American Psychiatric Association, 1700 18th Street N.W., Washington, D.C. 20009 (approx. $15.00).

Journal of Nervous and Mental Disorders, Williams & Wilkins Co., 428 East Preston Street, Baltimore, Maryland 21202 (approx. $35.00).

Child Psychiatry

American Journal of Orthopsychiatry, AOA Publications Sales Office, 49 Sheridan Avenue, Albany, New York 12210 (approx. $15.00).

Journal of the American Academy of Child Psychiatry, Yale University Press, 92A Yale Station, New Haven, Connecticut 06520 (approx. $20.00).

Reviews in Psychiatry

Annual Progress in Child Psychiatry and Child Development 1968, Brunner/Mazel, Inc., 64 University Place, New York, New York 10003. Reprint articles from American journals; tables of contents only.

Progress in Neurology and Psychiatry, Grune & Stratton, 111 Fifth Avenue, New York, New York 10003. Extensive subject index.

Yearbook of Psychiatry and Applied Mental Health 1970, Year Book Medical Publishers, Inc., 35 E. Wacker Dr., Chicago, Illinois 60601, Abstracts from journal articles; extensive subject index; author index.

Digests

Digest of Neurology and Psychiatry, The Institute of Living, 200 Retreat Avenue, Hartford, Connecticut 06106 (free).

Psychiatry Digest, Medical Digest Inc., 444 Frontage Road, Northfield, Illinois 60093 ($27.50/yr). A monthly summary of the world's psychiatry and neurology literature.

Other

Journal of Psychiatric Education, Human Sciences Press, 72 Fifth Avenue, New York, New York 10011.

Audio Cassettes

Audio Digest, Psychiatry, Audio-Digest Foundation, Dept. L.N., 762 1250 S. Glendale Avenue, Glendale, California 91205 (approx. $90.00).

Practical Reviews in Psychiatry, Educational Reviews, Inc., Box 582, Leeds, Alabama 35094 (approx. $110).

Indices

From time to time, a resident may wish to study a particular subject area in depth. The best source of help in this situation is several indices that are available in most university libraries for quick "manual" searches for articles on a particular subject or author's work. Practically speaking, these indices are available only through a librarian. They are of two basic types: The first type contains only reference citations for given subject areas or authors' works. The second type gives, in addition, an abstract or brief summary of the article cited.

A few of these indices are listed below.

Without Abstracts

Current Contents, Institute for Scientific Information, 325 Chestnut Street, Philadelphia, Pensylvania 19106. Covers life sciences, behavioral, social, educational sciences, etc.; listing of tables of contents of more than 1000 journals; weekly.

Index Medicus, U.S. National Library of Medicine, Bethesda, Maryland. Monthly bibliographic listing of references to current articles from approximately 2250 biomedical journals; author, title, subject approach to information and a separate bibliography of medical reviews.

Science Citation Index, Institute for Scientific Information, 325 Chestnut Street, Philadelphia, Pennsylvania 19106. Monthly; good journal coverage for psychiatry; references or name approach and subject approach to information.

Social Sciences Citation Index, Institute for Scientific Information, 325 Chestnut Street, Philadelphia, Pennsylvania 19106. Useful for finding material on a topic, for following an author's work, for finding later research based on an author's work, and for locating recent book reviews.

With Abstracts

Excerpta Medica: Section 32 Psychiatry, (Publ. Excerpta Medica Foundation), Elsevier North-Holland, Inc., 52 Vanderbilt Avenue, New York, New York 10017. Comprehensive coverage of all aspects of psychiatry.

Psychological Abstracts, American Psychological Association, 1200 Seventeenth Street, N.W., Washington, D.C. 20036. Covers over 900 journals and monographs; gives good coverage of the behavioral sciences; nonevaluative summaries of the world's literature in psychology and related disciplines; abstracts consist of descriptive summaries usually about 100 words in length; major access to psychological research; monthly; 2 annual volumes, each with a separate author and subject index.

Biological Abstracts, Bio-Sciences Information Service, 2100 Arch Street, Philadelphia, Pennsylvania 19103. Good for coverage of the biological basis for mental disorders.

Computerized Reference Services

If an extensive search is required in a short period of time, one must contact the librarian at the nearest health sciences library. The librarian will choose one or more international computer searches. Different data bases may be assessed depending on the area being searched. In North America, these searches usually cost between $5 and $25 and the data are usually available for your perusal within a week. Each type of search investigates a different "data base."

Psychological Abstracts Data Bases*

Computerized reference services (or "on-line services" for short) are a recent addition to the more traditional approach to library reference services—the manual search using printed indexes and abstracts. On-line services provide access to large subject-oriented indexes maintained on, and available through communication with, computers. Most of these data bases correspond to one or more printed sources. The computerized form allows for more efficient and flexible access to the information sought, and frequent updates ensure the currency of subject coverage. The result of an on-line search is a customized bibliography printed either on-line (more immediately available for use) or off-line (with re-

---

*This summary was compiled by Walter Zimmerman, The D. G. Weldon Library, University of Western Ontario, London, Onratio, Canada.

ceipt within one week, but significantly lower in cost than on-line printing). Some data bases such as *Psychological Abstracts* also have abstracts stored that may be printed as well. Access is accomplished by the specification and combination of index terms and other qualifiers (e.g., date, author affiliation) to provide a complete, but specific, bibliography.

Although the computer-aided bibliographic search involves a cost to the user, the benefits are numerous. The frustration and tedium of manual searches of printed indexes are avoided; the computer searches the entire listing (usually the equivalent of many volumes of the printed source) in a matter of minutes, retrieving relevant citations. Citations and abstracts may be printed out on-line or off-line, eliminating the effort of recording and maintaining manual files of pertinent citations. The multitopical approach available through on-line access to a variety of data bases allows for much greater ease in interdisciplinary searches, broad subject surveys, or cross-disciplinary information retrieval. In a study to determine comparative costs of manual vs. on-line searching, there was a five-to-one ratio in favor of the on-line search.

Because planning *before* the actual search takes place is critical to the success, an appointment should be made with the appropriate librarian–searcher. This allows for the development of an efficient and effective search strategy and ensures the librarian's undivided attention for the search. In most libraries, a search request form must be completed, providing an adequate subject outline, lists of terms, and information on limitations, expectations (i.e., a few very relevant citations or many relevant citations), scope, etc., to aid in the construction of an efficient and comprehensive search strategy. In the case of *Psychological Abstracts*, a thesaurus is available to simplify the selection of the proper index terms.* User presence during the on-line search is often encouraged so that the search results can be evaluated and the strategy modified to retrieve the most useful and appropriate number of references. Careful planning of the search reduces the cost as well, since costs are based on time spent on-line. Generally speaking, a number of categories are searchable. In *Psychological Abstracts*, these are author affiliation, author, title words, descriptors, identifiers, and abstracts. Once the search terms have been chosen, they can be combined with the operators "and," "or," and "not" to mirror your request. *This logic capability combined with a large number of searchable categories gives an advantage of specification considerably beyond the limits of manual selection.*

On-line searching is generally used for creating a one-time, retrospective bibliography on a specific topic. It can, however, be used in different ways. It can be used to quickly verify an elusive reference for interlibrary loan, and in fact, it is possible to order items on interlibrary loan via computer. It is also possible to purchase original copies of journal articles from over 5000 journals or theses from University Microfilms using an "Electronic Maildrop" feature. Finally, it is possible to keep current with a topic through an SDI (*S*elective *D*issemination of *I*nformation) profile. Once a month or every two months, newly indexed items matching your research needs will be sent to you for a modest fee.

*American Psychological Association: Thesaurus of Psychological Terms, 2nd ed., American Psychological Association, Washington, D.C., 1977.

Currently, *Psychological Abstracts* is the data base that, after Medline, is most beneficial to psychiatrists. It contains more than a quarter of a million references to psychology and related disciplines published since 1967 and grows at an annual rate of 25,000 references. Over 900 periodicals are scanned each year in producing the abstracts, as well as 1500 books, technical reports, and monographs. There are at present two commercial retrieval systems that provide on-line access to *Psychological Abstracts:* DIALOG and BRS. On both, the basic charge for computer time is $50 per hour and the cost for off-line printing is currently 10¢ per item with abstracts or 5¢ without abstracts on DIALOG and 15¢ per page with BRS. The cost of a typical search of six terms that might take 10 minutes and that would generate 25 references with abstracts would be $10.83. To this must sometimes be added a communications charge varying from the cost of a local telephone call to $20.00 per hour. A $20.00 hourly rate would add, in this example, $3.33, bringing the cost to $14.16. One would have saved hours of manual searching through *Psychological Abstracts*, however, and the results, if the search is well planned, should be better than results obtained by the traditional manual search method. If there is no library or other information facility available that can perform an on-line *Psychological Abstracts* search for you, you may write to the A.P.A. at 1700 18th St., N.W., Washington, D.C., 20036, and ask for PASAR (*PA Search And Retrieval*). They will perform your search and mail the results to you.

National Library of Medicine Data Bases*

In 1964, the National Library of Medicine, in Bethesda, Maryland, developed MEDLARS (*MEDical Literature Analysis and Retrieval System*), a computer-based system designed to achieve bibliographic access to biomedical journal information. In 1971, the National Library of Medicine developed a subset of MEDLARS into an on-line system accessible through telephone lines via Tymeshare nodes, and then gradually added more and more data bases.

It should be noted at the outset that the number of data bases is regularly being increased. In addition, the capabilities of individual data bases are constantly being expanded and/or changed. Here follows a description of the existing data bases and their present capabilities.

Medline

Thus, *Med*lars on-*line* (Medline) came into being. Its data bases now encompass the following: *Index Medicus, International Nursing Index, Index to Dental Literature.*

Coverage: Approximately 3000 journals from all over the world covering biomedical and related literature. Journals in peripheral areas are indexed only selectively as opposed to those directly related to the health sciences field, which are indexed from cover to cover. Example of selective indexing: "Abnormal or

*This summary was compiled by Mrs. Eva Borda, Research Librarian, The Health Sciences Centre Library, University of Western Ontario, London, Ontario, Canada.

absent β mRNAβ′ Ferrara and gene deletion in δβ thalassemia," *Nature* 263:471, 1976. This is an article that would be selected for indexing, whereas "Middle Pleistocene stratigraphy in southern East Anglia" on p. 492 of the same issue of *Nature* would definitely not be selected. The following is an example of the number of journals indexed selectively in some peripheral fields: biology, 98; botany, 5; engineering, 20; general science, 23; psychology and behavior, 90; sociology, 21.

Updating: The files are updated monthly and contain citations for the last two complete calendar years plus the current year.

Backfiles: It is possible, in a second stage, to gain access (off-line only) to information from 1966 onward.

Search Capability: A clear and concise statement of the user's request is necessary to enable librarians to formulate an appropriate search using a combination of annually updated *Index Medicus* terms (MeSH) and a free vocabulary, the latter being words taken from the author(s)' abstract and the title of the article and added to the regular *Index Medicus* vocabulary. Restriction of broad subjects is made possible by using any of 68 standard subheadings such as etiology, or diagnosis, or physiology, wherever applicable. Other possible restrictions are by language, geographic location, age, or form (e.g., abstracts or reviews), or by stating that certain aspects of a given subject are not required. (Example: "Emotional problems of handicapped but not mentally retarded children.") Searches may also be restricted by instructing the computer to retrieve citations only according to their primary aspects (e.g., a maximum of three subject headings under which an article is cross-referenced in the printed *Index Medicus*).

In case of a rather complex search, it might help to have the names of one to three authors who have written an article together on that particular subject within approximately the last two years. Correct spelling including initials is essential, or the computer will reject the names. A reference thus retrieved may then be displayed in "full"; i.e., in addition to the usual author(s), title, and source, all the key words and subheadings assigned to the article will be printed, enabling the analyst to formulate a search with regard to its specific subject content.

Citations may include various types of information. The standard form gives author(s), title, and source (journal title). A "Print full" command will display all major and minor descriptors used for indexing an article. One may also specify that the citation include the language of the original article, or one may request that an abstract (if available) be printed.

Medline was designed primarily to meet the immediate needs of researchers who are basically not interested in receiving unwieldy numbers of references. As opposed to MEDLARS, it is a fast retrieval system.

Limitations: It is, however, less valuable in retrieving the literature of very broad fields. The reasons are as follows:

1. Searches are limited to 25 search statements.
2. "And's," "or's," and "not's" may not be combined in one statement; they must be separated, which is a further restriction on the number of useful search statements.
3. On-line retrieval is limited to about 25–30 references, depending on the

length of the search formulation, because of the high cost of computer time.

4. Off-line printouts may contain a maximum of 300 citations.

One way of dealing with this problem is to use so-called "tree structures" and to instruct the computer in one statement to search simultaneously a whole string of related terms.

New Features: Because of the system's relative limitation with regard to searching subjects too broad to be included in one search, the National Library of Medicine has now introduced so-called "hedges." These are stored search fragments encompassing many cross categories. Thus, for example, a "hedge" such as "psychological aspects" added to "asthma" would retrieve all psychological, behavioral, and personality aspects, and it would include neuroses but not psychoses. At present, the following "hedges" are available (new ones will be added with time): "psychological aspects," "nutrition," "narcotics," "socioeconomic," "nursing," "immunological aspects," "cities," "developing and less-developed countries," and "epidemiology."

Another new feature is the appearance, in both the 1976 data base and the printed *Index Medicus*, of chapters taken from textbooks and published proceedings of international congresses. Examples are:

"Oculoplastic round table." pp. 167–79. Guibor, P. In: Guibor, P., and Smith, B., eds. Contemporary oculoplastic surgery. New York, Stratton, 1974. WW168 A5104c.

"Diagnosis of iron deficiency anemia." pp. 123–5. Crosby, W. H. In: Kief, H., *et al.*, eds. Iron metabolism and its disorders. Amsterdam, Excerpta Medica, 1975. W3 EX89, no. 366, 1975.

The "no. 366" in this latter example signifies the series called *Excerpta Medica International Congress Series.* For the convenience of the user, these book citations all end in a call number, i.e., the number by which the book may be found in most health sciences libraries arranged according to the National Library of Medicine's classification system.

SDI line

Includes the same fields as Medline and covers the same journals. The only differences are that only the latest indexed month may be accessed and that its sole purpose is to alert users to the most current indexed literature faster than the printed volume of *Index Medicus* reaches subscribers. In essence, it is a current awareness service.

Chemline

This is an on-line chemical dictionary file providing a mechanism whereby chemical substance names or name surrogates can be searched and retrieved. It contains records for all chemicals cited in the Toxline files, and should therefore *always* be searched before logging in Toxline.

Toxline

*Tox*icology information on-*line* is an interactive bibliographic retrieval system for toxicology consisting of seven subfiles: chemical–biological activities; toxicity bibliography; abstracts on health effect of environmental pollutants; *International Pharmaceutical Abstracts; Pesticides Abstracts*, formerly *Health Aspects of Pesticides Abstract Bulletin;* and environmental mutagen information center. On-line retrieval from this data base is a free-text-type searching of most words in titles, index fields, and abstracts. The on-line file contains approximately 400,000 records from 1971 forward. Older information (from 1965 on) is available off-line through Toxback.

Epilepsyline

Contains citations of articles abstracted by Excerpta Medica. The file contains references from 1947 to the present. This data base is supported by the National Institute of Neurological and Communicable Disorders and Stroke (U.S.).

Others

Other "special" lines are available. Consult your librarian.

Why Pay Money for a Computer Search When It May Also Be Done Manually?

The advantages of computerized information retrieval over searching the literature manually are:

Cross-Indexing: Any article appearing in the printed *Index Medicus* is cross-indexed under a maximum of three subject headings as opposed to the machine-readable file, in which up to 25 subject headings, plus textwords taken from the author(s)' abstract and other descriptors defining age groups, geographic locations, language, form, etc., are added by the indexer. In other words, information that needs the coordination of many subjects or aspects of it is found more readily by using a computer.

Current Updating: Files are updated monthly, long before the monthly issues of *Index Medicus* are printed and reach libraries, thus providing access to the latest indexed information.

Time Factor: Computer searches take minutes to do, whereas manually one may spend days to retrieve the same information—or less.

Costs

Charges are $5.00 per search. Backfiles (any or all of the period from 1966 to 1974) count as one search.

There is an additional charge for off-line printouts of 10¢ per page over and above 10 pages (or approximately 100 references).

Appendix C

Training Requirements*

American Medical Association: Excerpts from "Essentials of Approved Residencies"

21. Special Requirements for Residency Training in Psychiatry and Neurology

Residencies in Psychiatry and Neurology are offered separately.

Training in Psychiatry

I. INTRODUCTION

An approved residency program in psychiatry must demonstrate that it provides an educational experience of such quality and excellence as to assure that its graduates will possess mature clinical judgment and a high order of knowledge about the diagnosis, etiology, treatment, and prevention of all psychiatric disorders and the common neurological disorders. While residents cannot be expected to achieve in three years of training the highest possible degree of expertise in all of the diagnostic and treatment procedures used in psychiatry, those individuals who satisfactorily complete residency programs in psychiatry must be competent to render effective professional care to patients. Furthermore, they must have a keen awareness of their own strengths and limitations and of the necessity for continuing their own professional development.

The philosophy and organization of the residency program should make the resident aware that there are no short cuts to clinical competence, and no substitutes for hard individual study. The initiative and originality of all residents should be stimulated; their independence of mind promoted; and their ability to appraise critically the various schools of thought about human behavior should be encouraged.

---

*This appendix consists of paragraphs selected by the editor from the printed requirements for residency training for Australia, Canada, Great Britain, and the United States. The purpose of these excerpts is to provide a broad overview of the essentials for training in each of these countries. The resident must *not* rely on this appendix for anything more than a comparative overview. Each resident should obtain the complete regulations from the governing body in his or her country.

Both the didactic and clinical curriculum must provide a thorough and well balanced presentation of all of the generally accepted theories, schools of thought, and diagnostic or therapeutic procedures in the field of psychiatry and it must avoid indoctrinating residents in any single point of view. Thoughtful and informed appraisal of all of the major theories and viewpoints in psychiatry, together with a thorough grounding in the generally accepted facts, are fundamental to a sound professional education.

With rare exceptions, only those programs are eligible for approval which:

(1) Currently provide at least three years of residency education and as of July 1, 1977, provide four years of graduate education following receipt of the M.D. degree. (See regulations of the American Board of Psychiatry and Neurology.*)

(2) Are conducted under the sponsorship of a hospital which meets the General Requirements that apply to residency programs in all specialties as outlined in Sections I, II, III, and IV of Approved Residencies;

(3) Meet all of the Special Requirements of Residency Training in Psychiatry.

Under rare and unusual circumstances programs of either one year or two years duration may be approved, even though they do not meet all of the General Requirements or all of the Special Requirements for Psychiatry. Such one- or two-year programs will be approved only if they provide some highly specialized educational program of great excellence and outstanding value.

A minimum number (or "critical mass") of residents should be enrolled in a program at all times in order to insure the stimulating educational atmosphere that a good peer group provides. It is impossible to define exactly how many residents constitute the "critical mass" necessary to maintain the vitality of a program and insure a satisfactory educational climate. However, all programs must have at least two trainees in each year of training at all times if the program is to maintain full approval. Failure to recruit any new trainees for two consecutive years will result in disapproval of the program.

II. EDUCATIONAL PROGRAMS

Formal educational activity shall have high priority in the allotment of the resident's time and energies. The clinical responsibilities of residents must not infringe unduly on didactic educational activities and formal instruction.

However, the clinical care of patients is the heart of an adequate program since the chief objective of residency education is the development of a high order of clinical competence in its graduates. The attainment of this chief objective must not be attenuated by the participation of residents in other activities such as hos-

---

*The regulations of the American Board of Psychiatry and Neurology, referred to in (1) above, state that two patterns of training are acceptable:

1. Prior to entering an approved Psychiatry or Neurology training program, a physician must have completed one year of approved training after receiving the degree of Doctor of Medicine. This year of clinical experience should emphasize internal medicine or pediatrics or family practice.

2. A four-year training program in Psychiatry or in Neurology would be acceptable with the provision that at least one year be spent in an approved program providing direct responsibility for the general medical care of children and/or adults.

pital administration, ward management, the teaching of other hospital personnel, or research. Nevertheless, residents should obtain adequate and supervised experience in administration, ward management and teaching (hospital personnel, more junior residents, medical students, etc.).

Residents should also learn about research methodology, and develop the ability to appraise critically professional and scientific literature. Approved programs should provide opportunities for actual participation in clinical or basic research by residents, but, at the same time, research activity should not interfere with the development of clinical competence of residents.

Clinical and didactic teaching must be of sufficient breadth to insure that all residents become thoroughly acquainted with the major methods of diagnosis and treatment of mental illness which are recognized as significant both in this country and abroad.

Didactic instruction must be well organized, thoughtfully integrated, based on sound educational principles, and carried out on a regularly scheduled basis. In a progressive fashion it should expose residents to topics appropriate to their level of training. Systematically organized formal instruction (prepared lectures, seminars, assigned reading, etc.) must be an essential part of the residency. Staff meetings, clinical case conferences, journal clubs, and lectures by visitors are desirable adjuncts, but must not be used as substitutes for an organized didactic curriculum.

The faculty must provide instruction to help the resident develop the ability to interview patients effectively, to perform a comprehensive psychiatric examination and evaluation of mental status, to write histories clearly and in good detail, to produce a meaningful continuous record of the patient's illness, background and course of treatment, and to present or discuss the case in a lucid and thoughtful manner.

All residents must participate to a significant degree in regularly scheduled clinical case conferences in which the resident is responsible for presenting case material and discussing the relevant theoretical and practical issues. A significant proportion of the psychiatrists, psychologists, and other mental health professionals on the full-time faculty should attend these conferences as well as the residents and other personnel who have responsibility for the care of patients.

The curriculum must include adequate and systematic instruction in such basic sciences relevant to psychiatry and neurology, and neuroanatomy, neurophysiology, neuropathology, neurochemistry, pharmacology, genetics, psychopathology, nosology, psychodynamics, and sufficient material from the social and behavioral sciences (such as psychology, anthropology, sociology) to help the resident understand the importance of economic, ethnic, social and cultural factors in mental health and mental illness. The curriculum must also provide a thorough grounding in medical ethics and in the history of psychiatry and its relation to the evolution of modern medicine.

The clinical portion of the curriculum must provide experience in:

(1) Psychiatric care of adults, children, and adolescents in both inpatient and outpatient settings;
(2) Clinical psychophysiology or psychosomatic medicine;

(3) Psychiatric consultation or liaison psychiatry involving patients hospitalized on other clinical services such as pediatrics, medicine, surgery, obstetrics and gynecology;

(4) Hospital emergency room (or some equivalent experience in emergency care);

(5) Crisis intervention;

(6) Community psychiatry;

(7) Neurology; and

(8) Forensic psychiatry.

The clinical services must be organized so that residents have basic responsibility for the care of a significant proportion of all patients assigned to them, and so that they have an appropriate amount of supervision by the staff. Residents must have the major responsibility for the diagnosis and treatment of a reasonable number of patients suffering from all of the major categories of psychiatric illness and ample experience in the diagnosis and management of the more common neurological disorders. They must have experience in the care of patients of both sexes, patients of various ages from childhood to senility, and patients from a wide variety of ethnic, social, and economic backgrounds.

Clinical training must include regularly scheduled individual supervision and teaching rounds. In addition, all programs should provide some scheduled time for residents to pursue individually chosen electives.

The amount and type of basic responsibility for patient care that a resident assumes must increase as the resident advances in training. Responsibility must at all times be commensurate with the resident's abilities and clinical competence.

The training program must include a significant amount of time spent in the care of hospitalized patients. It is recommended that residents devote at least one-third of their resident experience to work with hospitalized patients. It is undesirable for a program to devote more than two-thirds of a resident's time to the care of hospitalized patients.

The number of patients in the care of a resident at any one time must be sufficiently small to permit adequate study and treatment of each patient on an individual basis. At any given time the resident should have primary clinical responsibility for no more than approximately 20 inpatients.

Clinical assignments for residents must provide experience in the continuous care of a significant number of patients (approximately ten) for at least a year or more. A portion (approximately five) of the patients for whom the resident has responsibility for such continuous care must be patients suffering from chronic psychotic illnesses.

A significant amount of the resident's clinical work must involve active collaboration with psychologists, psychiatric nurses, social workers and other professional and para-professional mental health personnel.

Diagnostic skills in psychiatry should include active familiarity with all the generally accepted psychometric techniques and instruments. A reasonable amount of the resident's clinical work must involve the use of the more common psychological test procedures sufficient to give the resident an understanding of the clinical usefulness of these procedures, and the correlation of psychological test findings with clinical data. Under the supervision of a qualified clinical psychologist residents should have some experience in the administration, scoring, and interpretation of the psychological tests in most common use. Some of the experience residents have in administering psychological tests should be with their own patients.

Through the didactic and clinical curriculum, the program must provide all residents with sound instruction and clinical experience in neurology. The psychiatry resident must be able to obtain a thorough history regarding neurological disease, perform a competent neurological examination, make a differential neurological diagnosis, and, under supervision, plan and carry out the treatment of the common, clinically important neurological diseases. This requires a substantial and specific assignment during which each resident has clinical responsibility for the diagnosis and treatment of neurological patients. This requirement is particularly important because of the natural blend of the manifestations of psychiatric illness and neurological disease, and the frequent complications of one by the other.

The curriculum must involve a significant number of clinical conferences and didactic seminars in which psychiatric faculty members collaborate with neurologists, internists, and colleagues from other medical specialties.

The clinical training in community psychiatry should include experience in a community mental health center or some equivalent setting, and consultation to at least one community agency such as a school, court, or police department.

Training in forensic psychiatry must involve more than solely didactic instruction. It should include supervised clinical experiences such as consultative work with judges, attorneys, police, probation officers, and other professionals in the legal field, and wherever possible, actual experience in courtroom testimony.

All programs must contain substantial didactic education and supervised clinical experience in the inpatient and outpatient treatment of children and adolescents. The resident should gain a thorough understanding of the biological, psychological, social, economic, ethnic and family factors that significantly influence physical and psychological development in infancy, childhood, and adolescence.

III. DIRECTOR OF RESIDENCY PROGRAM AND PARTICIPATING FACULTY*

Each residency program must be under the direction of a fully qualified psychiatrist whose primary responsibility on the staff is to maintain an educational program of excellence. The training director should be responsible for maintaining:

(1) A process for selecting as residents physicians who are personally and professionally suited for training in psychiatry;

(2) Well-planned and systematic educational activities of excellent quality;

---

*The official regulations should be consulted for further paragraphs amplifying these sections. Only the initial paragraphs have been included here, and all of Section IV, "Clinical and Educational Facilities and Resources," has been omitted.

(3) Regular and systematic evaluation of the progress of each resident, including complete records of evaluations containing explicit statements on the resident's progress and his major strengths and weaknesses;

(4) A program of regularly scheduled meetings with each resident, of sufficient frequency, length and depth to insure that the resident is continually aware of the quality of his progress toward attainment of professional competence;

(5) Procedures for helping the resident obtain appropriate help for significant personal or professional problems;

(6) Procedures for the proper and judicious resolution of problems that occur when a resident's performance does not meet required standards. These procedures should be fair to the resident, the patient under his care, the training program, and to the profession; and

(7) A written record of the educational responsibilities of all staff and faculty members (whether full-time or part-time) who participate directly in the education of residents, including the nature, frequency, and amount of time involved in the teaching activity of each.

Child Psychiatry

There is a basic core of training necessary for competence in Child Psychiatry, no matter what the eventual area of practice, be it in community child guidance clinics, in university teaching centers, in research, public health, administration, private practice, etc. The basic essential of sound training is a practical, well-rounded learning experience in clinical Child Psychiatry. This training should take place in a medically-directed child psychiatry facility.

The training program should offer a well-balanced patient load, supervised treatment, and diagnostic and consultative work with children and their parents. The supervisors of training should be competent, experienced child psychiatrists, The clinical material with which the fellow-in-training has experience should provide not only a wide range of problems of varying types and degrees of severity but also diversification of age, social-economic status, and sex. Training should include experience in working collaboratively with psychiatric social workers and clinical psychologists. There should be provision for co-operative consultative work with medical facilities for children. There should be opportunity for consultative work with various community child-care agencies. During the training experience, there should be practical and didactic teaching. The areas covered should include the practice of Child Psychiatry with diagnosis and differential diagnosis, psychiatric treatment methods including psychotherapy and collaborative treatment, normal and pathological development, and the literature of the field.

Whenever feasible, the career Child Psychiatrist should receive a block of two years of training in Child Psychiatry following his two years in general psychiatry. However, to achieve greater flexibility in the sequence of training for the career Child Psychiatrist, and to assist in recruitment, the training experience for a career Child Psychiatrist may be initiated in any of the three years of General

Psychiatric residency training provided that the training be full-time, a block of time spent at any one time is not less than six months, and that if a six-month block is chosen it be followed at another time by not less than an 18-month block of full-time training in Child Psychiatry; two separate 12-month full-time blocks in Child Psychiatry may also be chosen.

ACKNOWLEDGMENT

Special thanks are given to the American Medical Association for permission to reprint this material.

The Royal College of Physicians and Surgeons of Canada: "Specialty Training Requirements in Psychiatry"

General Objectives

The objective of the graduate training program in psychiatry is the training of a medical specialist who is expert in the application of relevant, medical, surgical, biological, psychological, and social factors to the diagnosis, treatment, and management of psychiatric disorders. At the end of training, the graduate must be capable of assuming therapeutic management in the most effective and efficient manner. It is thus necessary for the trainee to have adequate definable knowledge, skills, and attitudes that will enable the fulfilment of the above general objectives. This will require, as well, that the psychiatric specialist acquire skills in working collaboratively with other health workers to provide psychiatric health services that are comprehensive and readily available. In addition, the psychiatrist should have special sensitivity to the consequences of such factors as poverty, discrimination, violence, and disrupted family life.

All postgraduate trainees in psychiatry in Canada must register with a university and plan their training programs in collaboration with the director of the residency program in psychiatry. Trainees moving to another approved centre for other training are urged to do so under the auspices of their original or "home" program. It is strongly advised, however, that the trainee complete at least two years (see below) of residency training in one program.

Postgraduate training in psychiatry involves a minimum of four years approved training after the general internship (see "1. Internship" below). Three of these years must be spent in a clinical psychiatric experience, and at least two of these three years must be spent in an intensive learning situation that provides the necessary basic clinical experience and related didactic instruction. The additional two years of resident training, also under university direction, provide a wider choice for the trainee (see Section 2(b) of the Training Requirements). This will allow a resident to complete two years of training in a subspecialty area, such as child psychiatry, within the four years of residency training.

The basic clinical training requirements described above, which will encompass at least two years of the program, must include a minimum of one year of a general hospital type of experience on the psychiatric services of a hospital central to the university program, with experience in both the inpatient and outpatient or ambulatory care units. The hospital must offer, in addition to its ordinary outpatient activities, opportunities to participate in community medicine and crisis management. There should also be a learning experience in psychosomatic medicine including consultation and liaison experiences with opportunities available to play a direct role in the diagnostic workup and treatment plan of patients with more complicated medical and psychiatric problems. Opportunities to work with and learn from other medical disciplines and with other non-psychiatric professionals who are part of the psychiatric health team (see 2(a) below) should be available.

The basic training program must also include six months, and preferably one year, of experience and study devoted entirely to the comprehensive care, of children, adolescents, and their families (see 2(a) below).

The basic training program must further include at least six months, and preferably one year, of experience in the comprehensive care and rehabilitation of both acute and long-term psychotic patients. During this experience the trainee must receive instruction and supervision in the proper utilization of long-term treatment techniques as well as gain experience in dealing with the medical-legal problems peculiar to this type of patient. This training in the management of long-stay patients may be taken concurrently with other parts of the basic training program.

The areas of skill and knowledge that must be covered in the didactic supervised clinical experiences before basic training can be considered complete will include:

> basic patterns of disease
> historical trends in psychiatry
> normal and abnormal psychosexual development
> contributions of the biological sciences
> contributions of the psychological sciences
> contributions of the socio-cultural sciences
> child and adolescent psychiatry
> mental retardation
> genetics
> theories of personality and psychopathology
> psychiatric assessment
> psychiatric emergencies
> psychophysiological disorders
> psychosocial reactions to illness
> psychiatric syndromes
> methods of treatment
>> psychopharmacology and other biological therapies
>> behavior modification
>> the psychotherapies
>> social therapies
> community and administrative psychiatry
> geriatric psychiatry
> forensic psychiatry
> psychiatric research and research methods.

During the training there should be a minimum of two years of an adequately supervised psychotherapy experience with adult patients as well as psychotherapy experience with children and adolescents.

Applicants who take their psychiatric training outside of Canada must fulfil the training requirements described above.

Eligibility to sit the written part of the examinations, a multiple choice examination, is achieved after the satisfactory completion of at least two years of the specialty training requirements in an approved Canadian training program, with the approval of the Canadian training program director. This part of the training will be organized and integrated by the supervising program director of the department of psychiatry as the "core program" of the department in relation to the total specialty training requirements.

1. Internship

Graduates of Canadian or United States medical schools who have had an undergraduate clinical clerkship (see "General Information," Section 5) may fulfil one of the required years of resident training in psychiatry by taking one year of approved straight internship in psychiatry in a fully approved resident training program or take one year of approved straight internship in medicine (preferably including neurology and psychiatry) in a fully approved resident training program. All other graduates must complete an approved internship of at least one year's duration *in addition* to the four years of specialty training described below.

2. Specialty Training Requirements

Four years of approved training. This period must include:

a) Three years of approved residency training in clinical psychiatry, which must include:
   i) At least two years of basic clinical training, including at least one year of a general hospital type of experience in a hospital that is central to the university program, as stated above in the general objectives.
   ii) At least six months, and preferably one year, of experience within the two years of basic clinical training devoted entirely to the psychiatric care of children, adolescents, the mentally retarded, and their families.
   iii) At least six months, and preferably one year, in the study and comprehensive care of psychotic and long-stay patients. This may be concurrent with other basic training.

b) In addition to the above basic clinical and didactic learning experiences in psychiatry, the remaining year may include:
   i) One year of further approved training as outlined under Section 2(a) at an increased level of responsibility, such as in a senior or chief resident capacity.
   ii) Six months or one year of approved resident training in a psychiatric subspecialty. In conjunction with Section 2(a), this will allow up to two years of training in a subspecialty.

iii) Six months or one year in the full-time study of a related basic science, such as neuro-anatomy, neurophysiology, psychology, or sociology, in a department acceptable to the Royal College and recommended by the program director in psychiatry.

iv) Six months or one year in an approved residency training program in internal medicine, family medicine, neurology, pediatrics, or other branch of medicine related to psychiatry.

v) One year of resident training in an approved mental hospital or similar unit.

vi) Six months or one year of approved training or research, relevant to the objectives of psychiatry and acceptable to the director of the training program and to the College, at a hospital or university centre in Canada or abroad.

(Adopted June 1977)

(These training requirements apply to those who begin creditable training on or after July 1, 1978.)

Specific Requirements and Guidelines for Accreditation of Specialty Training Programs in Psychiatry

The requirements and guidelines that apply to all specialty training programs are set out fully in the two companion booklets:

(1) "General Information Concerning Accreditation of Specialty Training Programs"
(2) "In-training Evaluation Systems in Postgraduate Medical Education: Accreditation Requirements and Guidelines."

I. The Integrated Program

An accredited training program must provide opportunities for trainees to achieve the educational objectives in psychiatry that are outlined in the blue booklet: "Specialty Training Requirements in the Medical and Laboratory Specialties."

The overall training program must provide, through the facilities of the university and the participating institutions, the following:

1. Adequate inpatient, consultation and ambulatory care facilities for the clinical investigation, treatment, and follow-up psychiatric patients, with a sufficient number and variety of patients, including children, to provide opportunities for training and experience over the full range of psychiatry and associated fields.

2. An emergency department and intensive care units for experience in critical care.

3. A sufficient number of qualified teaching staff to supervise the trainees and provide teaching in the basic sciences related to psychiatry.

4. A coordinated educational program in psychiatry that provides graduated increases in trainee responsibility as experience is gained in the manage-

ment of psychiatric patients. The training must include responsibility, under supervision, for the total care of the patient, including the physical condition.

5. Consultative experience on inpatients in the clinical teaching units of other disciplines and on outpatients.

II. The Institutional Components of the Program

1. The institution, if an adult or children's hospital, must, with rare exceptions, be participating in Royal College approved specialty training programs in medicine or pediatrics, surgery, pathology, and radiology. Normally, it should also be engaged in teaching undergraduate medicine, including psychiatry.
2. The psychiatric service must be organized into one or more formal clinical teaching units, each with an adequate number of patients available for teaching and administered by a chief-of-service to whom the senior resident is directly responsible.
3. There must be an outpatient department or alternative facilities for the provision of experience in the management and follow-up of psychiatric outpatients.

December, 1976

ACKNOWLEDGMENT

Special thanks are given to the Royal College of Physicians and Surgeons of Canada for permission to reprint this material.

The Royal Australian and New Zealand College of Psychiatrists: Excerpts from "By-Laws and Booklet for the Information of Candidates, 1978"

Part Two: R.A.N.Z.C.P. Examination for Membership

Part Two A: By-Laws

Applicable to those who begin training after 1st January, 1978.*

1. A candidate for entry to the College shall make application on prescribed forms, to attend Sections I and II of the examination, at the relevant times, in order to qualify for such entry. He or she will be required to produce evidence of:

(a)   entry on the current Register of Medical Practitioners of a State of the Commonwealth of Australia or of the Dominion of New Zealand or of some other country, state or dependency approved by the General Council for the purpose of this By-law;

(b)   having spent one (1) year as a Resident Medical Officer (or in an

*Part Two B, for candidates who have begun training prior to December 31, 1977, has not been included here. This part may be obtained from the College.

equivalent position in New Zealand) in a General Hospital approved
by the Board of Censors;

(c) A. at the time of application for Section I of the examination has spent
not less than three (3) years and six (6) months continuous training
in full-time psychiatric practice which shall occur in facilities accredited by the College and include:

    (i) not less than four (4) hours clinical supervision per week for a
minimum of three (3) years and not less than forty (40) weeks
in each of those years. At least one of these four hours per week
shall be individual supervision. In all years, experience should
concentrate on male and female patients suffering from acute
and chronic psychiatric disorders. An intensive shorter "block"
period of supervision is not recognised as equivalent in hours.
Time involved in formal psychotherapy training, and time spent
in seminars devoted to discussion of theoretical issues, shall be
in addition to the above requirements.

    (ii) not less than 20% of the time in family, developmental and re-
lated aspects of psychiatry (this includes child psychiatry *but
must not be exclusively in child psychiatry units*).

    (iii) a period of six (6) months experience in liaison psychiatric whilst
in full time attendance at the psychiatric department of a general hospital or an agreed equivalent.

    (iv) a period of six (6) months' full-time attendance at a psychiatric
hospital specialising in the treatment and rehabilitation of acute
and chronic patients.

(c) B. Prior to presentation for Section II of the examination the candidate
must have undertaken a further period of training of a fifth (5th) year
which may consist of experience in general psychiatry or one or more
of a number of electives by prior agreement with the Board of Censors, and which must take place in facilities approved for that purpose by the College. These electives will include child and family psychiatry, forensic psychiatry, administrative psychiatry, community
psychiatry, research, psychotherapy, adolescent psychiatry, neuropsychiatry, etc.

The candidate cannot apply for Section II before the latter part of
the fifth (5th) year.

2. The Board of Censors may, at its discretion, accept a candidate for the
membership examination if it is satisfied that his experience in all essential aspects is equivalent to that set out in the previous paragraph.

3. Section I of the examination for which the candidate applies on form A,
provides the following: at least three (3) months prior to the date of the written
examination, the candidate shall submit to the Board of Censors five (5) case histories, each history to be not less than 2,000 words or more than 8,000 words in
length. Each history shall describe the illness, diagnosis, investigation and treatment of a patient who has been in the candidate's personal care and is to be accompanied by a note from a Fellow or Member of the College on the full-time

or part-time staff of the unit in which the patient was studied, certifying that to the best of the knowledge and belief of such Fellow or Member that history is the candidate's own work.

4. The patients reported shall be:

(a) one patient with an acute psychiatric disorder, admitted for the first time to an in-patient psychiatric unit;

(b) one patient seen in the long stay wards of a psychiatric hospital; or a patient with a chronic psychiatric disorder in some other forms of care;

(c) one patient less than fourteen (14) years old, and perhaps the patient's family;

(d) one patient or family treated by psychotherapy for a minimum of approximately fifty (50) sessions.

N.B.: In exceptional circumstances, the Board will accept more than one case where this is required to make up the fifty (50) sessions.

(e) one patient with known organic disease of the central nervous system related to his psychiatric illness.

5. Only those candidates who, in the opinion of the Board of Censors, present case histories which are considered to be at a satisfactory level, will be permitted to attempt the written examination.

6. If the case histories are considered to be of a satisfactory standard, but the candidate subsequently fails in any portion of the examination, he will not be required to present these case histories on any future occasion.*

Part Three: Accreditation

The need for accreditation of training programs and teaching units has been recognised by Postgraduate Medical Colleges throughout Australia. The Royal Australian and New Zealand College of Psychiatrists is accrediting the training of individuals, not teaching institutions.

The Board of Accreditation of the College will introduce the accreditation procedures in stages over the next few years. As accreditation is developed, additional procedures will be introduced. In 1978 the first stage will be implemented: the accreditation of training programs in adult general psychiatry.

The Board of Accreditation will require an undertaking by the Director or Superintendent of teaching institutions to offer *each trainee* in adult general psychiatry the type of supervision, experience and facilities as laid down in the regulations governing accreditation. This undertaking will be required from 1st January 1978.

At the end of the trainee's period in adult general psychiatry, the Director or Superintendent of the teaching institution and the trainee will certify that the regulations of the Board of Accreditation have been satisfied. This certification will be on the prescribed form, Accreditation Form C.

---

*Paragraphs 7 through 13 have been omitted. They apply specifically to the examinations, rather than to the essentials of training.

Regulations Concerning Accreditation

Each unit seeking to be accredited, other than as a special unit, shall certify in advance to the Board of Accreditation that for a period of one year, it will supply a particular nominated candidate with the following services and experiences:

1. Not less than four hours clinical supervision per week, for not less than forty weeks in that year. At least one of the four hours per week shall be individual supervision. Experience shall concentrate on male and female patients suffering from acute and chronic psychiatric disorders. An intensive shorter "block" period of supervision is not recognised as equivalent in hours. Time involved in formal psychotherapy, behaviour therapy or other specialised therapeutic techniques shall be in addition to the above requirements, as shall time spent in seminars devoted to the discussion of theoretical issues. The essence of each session is that it shall be clinical and concerned with patients.

2. These sessions of clinical supervision shall be scheduled, and conducted by Clinical Supervisors, individually specified in the application submitted by the institution seeking accreditation.

3. A Clinical Supervisor shall be a Fellow or Member of the College. Until, but not including the year 1981, these duties may be performed by any psychiatrist whose qualifications are approved by the Board of Accreditation. Thereafter the Board will approve supervision by a psychiatrist who is not a Fellow or Member of the College only in exceptional circumstances, and for a limited period.

4. During the time that the candidate is on duty, there shall be a Clinical Supervisor available to him for consultation about clinical problems.

5. One of the candidate's Clinical Supervisors shall be designated his Clinical Tutor. He shall be responsible for supervising the candidate's clinical work generally, and for ensuring that it is of satisfactory standard. This particularly includes keeping proper clinical notes of each case. At the end of the year he shall certify that the candidate's clinical work was satisfactory.

6. The institution shall warrant that during the candidate's training, there shall be a clear line of responsibility from a particular patient, to a particular psychiatrist or medical officer.

8. The institution shall warrant that the range and nature of psychiatric disorders to which the candidate is exposed in the course of his training is not greatly different from what might be expected in any unit offering a general psychiatric in-patient service. The notion is that the in-patient population encountered by the candidate should reflect prevalence of psychiatric disorder in the general community, rather than a distribution determined by research, special interests or other factors.

9. Provided that there is compliance with these regulations it is permissible for a candidate's year of training to take place in more than one institution. For example, a candidate employed at a city hospital might spend part of his time seconded to a country hospital. In this case, the onus of ensuring that there is compliance with the regulations rests with the primary employer.

10. At the end of the year, the accredited institution shall certify that the candidate presented himself for mandatory periods of supervision, and that his clinical work reached an acceptable standard. This is in addition to the certificate given by the Clinical Tutor.

11. Units which fail to meet the agreed requirements in one year shall not be eligible for accreditation in the succeeding year, unless there have been special extenuating circumstances, and unless the Board can be satisfied that these circumstances can be remedied.

12. At the end of the year the candidate shall certify that he received the services and conditions specified above.

13. Candidates who certify falsely that they have received the specified supervision and facilities when they did not receive them, shall not be considered to have received a year of accredited training in that year. Applications for further training will be considered only if the Board is satisfied that there have been special extenuating circumstances.

14. Each institution obtaining accreditation for its program will be required to pay $20.00 per annum (once only, not per candidate) being a contribution towards such clerical, administrative and inspection expenses as may be necessary.

Board of Accreditation
JOHN ELLARD
Chairman

The Australian and New Zealand College of Psychiatrists, Section of Child Psychiatry: Minimal Training Standard for Child Psychiatrists (Amended 1971)

1. In keeping with an approved motion at the Annual General Meeting of the Section of Child Psychiatry in October 1970, the Section of Child Psychiatry recommends that in principle the certification by the College of child psychiatrists, be provisional on the candidate possessing membership of the Australian and New Zealand College of Psychiatrists (or its equivalent) and on having worked for two years in an approved Child Psychiatry Unit.

2. Structure of Training Programme:
   (a) Minimum training period of two years, full time.
   (b) This period to be a flexible structured "apprenticeship" leading to appropriate certification by the College.
   (c) Continuous supervision throughout the course by a recognized child psychiatrist in approved institutions. This should be both an overall control of the candidate's activities, and a more detailed involvement in the candidate's contacts with various aspects of child psychiatry by appropriately experienced supervisors.

3. Content of Programme:
   (a) Experience in:
      - Diagnostic assesment
      - Direct management, including psychotherapy, physical treatment, intervention in family problems
      - Consultation and indirect management

   of

      - Acute and chronic psychiatric problems (inpatient and outpatient general child psychiatry)

- Mental Retardation
- Anti-social behaviour and delinquency
- Paediatric problems, including physical handicaps, rehabilitation, emotional problems of institutionalization
- Developmental delay or deviation
- Psychosomatic illness
- Neurological disorders
- Educational problems
- Psychiatric problems of adolescents

(b) More formal "instruction" by lectures, seminars, case conferences, etc. to cover:
- Normal child development from infancy to adolescence
- The Family—structure and relationships: Social and Community aspects
- Common developmental reactions and deviations in children—reaction to physical illnesses, situational reactions, neurotic and psychotic reactions
- Children with character disorders and personality disorders
- Organic illness in children, specific difficulties, e.g., sensory, cerebral palsy, multiple handicapped children
- Psychophysiologic reactions
- Mental Retardation
- Delinquency, work of the Children's Court
- Problems of the Adolescent
- Psychological and psychosocial methods
- Aspects of research
- Experience in teaching and administration
- Child Welfare problems
- Prevention and Research in relation to children's mental health
- Professional Roles and relationships of the child psychiatrist.

4. Approval of courses and training units will be by Officers of the College, appointed by the Council.

ACKNOWLEDGMENT

Special thanks are given to the Royal Australian and New Zealand College of Psychiatrists for permission to reprint this material.

The Royal College of Psychiatrists (London, England): Excerpts from "Educational Programmes for Trainees in Psychiatry"

The Royal College of Psychiatrists can only lay down guidelines for trainees in psychiatry because:
(a) no single training programme can be acceptable for the varied activities that consultant psychiatrists might undertake

(b) the service demands of hospitals where training is carried out are varied
(c) trainees differ in their abilities and their medical experience before commencing psychiatric training.

This guide is aimed mainly at trainees but it is hoped that it will also be of assistance to Clinical Tutors in giving advice to their junior colleagues. The current programmes of approval by the Royal College of Psychiatrists of hospitals for training will also take into account the College's general approval of broad but integrated patterns of training that may include several hospitals.

At the end of the three years' general professional training the aim for most trainees will be attempts at the M.R.C.Psych. Examinations and promotion to Senior Registrar grade at approximately the same time.

Candidates for the Membership Examination must have passed the Preliminary Test which would normally be taken after about one year's recognised training.

Basic Clinical Experience

The three years of training that is required for the M.R.C.Psych. Examination can be occupied in a variety of ways and in more than one hospital or group of hospitals. Much of this period of training should involve the supervised experience of the assessment and management of patients of all ages suffering from disorders representative of the whole range of psychiatric practice.

Some trainees, at present and in the future, will be mainly based on hospitals or institutions catering for one of the recognised sub-specialties, for example, mental handicap or forensic psychiatry (within the prison service). Others may be working almost entirely in general psychiatric hospitals or the psychiatric units of District General Hospitals and have little or no experience of these sub-specialties, nor of others such as child psychiatry and psychotherapy. It is not possible to lay down clear-cut maximum or minimum periods of experience in these sub-specialties. However, as a guide it is suggested, for example, that trainees working mainly in hospitals for the mentally handicapped for the full three years before taking the M.R.C.Psych. Examination should be able to spend at least one-half of their time acquiring clinical experience and formal training in other branches of psychiatry and related disciplines. Proportionately less time need be spent in general psychiatry if the trainee spends only 1 or 2 years in hospitals or units caring mainly for patients of one of the sub-specialties.

On the other hand, trainees primarily based on a general psychiatric hospital should have the opportunity of learning about the sub-specialties not only by formal lectures, demonstrations and seminars, but also by practical clinical experience in at least some if not all of them. In particular, experience in child psychiatry, mental handicap and psychotherapy, should be regarded as essential. Owing to the current lack of adequate teaching facilities in child psychiatry in many areas of the country, even minimally acceptable standards may still be unobtainable. The time spent in child psychiatry may be in a full-time block of, say, three to six months, or, preferably, a longer part-time assignment so that trainees can see a variety of children and their families for diagnostic assessment and a few for treatment. The essential criterion for the training is adequate supervision by a consultant child psychiatrist working in a fully equipped and well-staffed clinic, with access to the educational as well as the medical milieux in which child psychiatrists operate.

Training in psychotherapy poses special problems as continuity and experience with particular patients over at least two years is essential. Thus, though in general it is desirable to obtain experience at more than one hospital or to move around within a group of hospitals, every effort should be made to maintain continuity of training for individual and group psychotherapy. If possible, trainees under the supervision of psychotherapists should treat a few individual patients, manage at least one group and have experience of wards run as "therapeutic communities."

Experience in Subjects Related to Psychiatry

There are several branches of medicine and several basic sciences with a clear relationship to psychiatry, and in these up to one year of special experience in approved posts may be counted for the M.R.C.Psych. Examination. This experience may be taken at any time during the three years prior to entering the Membership Examination.

Full-time study in non-clinical fields, such as, for example, psychology, sociology, epidemiology, for up to one year would be welcome, provided that there is some link with clinical psychiatric work.

Full-time clinical research in any topic related to psychiatry or disciplines near it, such as neurophysiology or sociology, will receive particularly sympathetic consideration as part of general professional training. Candidates may offer a dissertation based on personal research in lieu of the essay paper in the Membership Examination. Notice of such intention must be given at least one year prior to the examination and further details are available from the College.

After about three years when the M.R.C.Psych. Examination may have been attempted, if not passed, and a Senior Registrar post obtained, trainees may have periods of special experience, perhaps in a sub-specialty. The organisation of such experience is outside the scope of these recommendations and will be the subject of further reports. However, if, for some reason, experience in special fields such as, for example, child psychiatry or psychotherapy, was lacking in the initial three years, efforts should be made to obtain the necessary familiarity with these subjects.

All trainees should turn to their local Clinical Tutor for advice at every stage of their training career. The tutors and trainees may apply to the Dean or Court of Electors for further advice.

Educational Programmes in Practical Psychiatry

Mere contact with psychiatric patients in psychiatric hospitals and community services is not sufficient training and the following opportunities for learning should also be provided:

(i) Regular presentation of patients clerked by the trainee to a Consultant or Senior Registrar in the setting of a ward round or a clinical conference. The teacher will aim at inculcating the principles of history-taking, physical and mental examination of the patient, diagnostic formulation, patient treatment and rehabilitation, including physical and psychotherapeutic methods and the use of social services.

(ii) Attendance at clinical conferences where there can be an exchange of views between several members of the senior staff and where the emphasis is on teaching. There should be a minimum of 25 attendances each year.

(iii) Participation in seminars and/or journal clubs (at least 10 a year).

(iv) Especially when caring for out-patients, the trainee will be taught how to ensure continuing care for his patients by working in liaison with general practitioners, psychiatric social workers, nurses and other colleagues, all of whom should be encouraged to play an active part in most teaching sessions.

(v) Courses in clinical psychology, both diagnostic and therapeutic, should be provided, if possible by clinical psychologists. Such instruction should include the use of intelligence and other psychological tests applicable to the investigation of psychiatric problems.

(vi) Individual and group psychotherapy, as mentioned above, should be carried out under the supervision of psychotherapists. The first emphasis should be on the understanding of the doctor/patient relationship and the principles of group methods, including the therapeutic community.

Role of Clinical Tutors

The Clinical Tutors in charge of teaching programmes based on one or more hospitals have two main roles. The first is directed towards the guidance of trainees, as already mentioned; the second is to organise and administer a teaching programme. The former involves regular personal contact with the trainees in their group of hospitals. The latter might include the organisation of individual seminars, the setting of essays, topics for research etc. Only in this way can the tutor provide adequate confidential reports if these are needed by the Royal College of Psychiatrists. He can also testify that the candidate's clinical experience fulfills the regulations for the M.R.C.Psych. Examination. In this way he can also act as one of the candidate's sponsors for the Membership Examination.

As regards the organisation of the teaching programmes, the Clinical Tutor should act as a close link between his hospital group and the related University Departments of Psychiatry, and the post-graduate activities of the Royal College of Psychiatrists.

There are also important functions of Clinical Tutors in relation to the teaching of trainees other than in psychiatry. In certain places, a second Clinical Tutor may, for example, have to be appointed to deal with the psychiatric training of general practitioners, though their programmes should be closely co-ordinated with the full psychiatric training.

Clinical Tutors also have special responsibilities towards other mental health workers, especially nurses, social workers etc., whose training should as far as possible be in common with psychiatric trainees so that they get to know each other.

Roles of the University Departments of Psychiatry

University Departments of Psychiatry are being increasingly involved with teaching programmes though the actual administrative arrangements are determined by local conditions. The fullest contact with the University Teachers should be ensured by allowing the maximum number of visits by the trainees (two weekly sessions in term time) tot he Psychiatric Departments of the post-graduate centres under the recommendations of the Health Department HM(67) and SHM 29/67. These contacts should, however, be supplemented by the University Teachers regularly visiting the peripheral hospitals to give lectures, chair conferences etc.

The University Departments must supplement both the basic education and the clinical teaching provided through the Clinical Tutors in the other hospitals. These deficiencies are most likely to appear in:

(a) sub-specialties within psychiatry, especially psychotherapy;
(b) subjects related to psychiatry, including neurology and basic sciences such as neurophysiology, and above all the sciences of psychology and sociology.

In both cases the University Departments will be able to call upon the collaboration of other consultants and University Departments in the teaching of these subjects. The University Departments have a particular role to play in the initiation of guidance of research and in giving advice to trainees about the preparation of M.D. theses.

It is desirable for every trainee to spend some time in a University Department of Psychiatry. This could be to obtain special experience in any clinical field or in a related basic science, or for the purpose of carrying out a piece of research. Rotation or secondment schemes are available for some trainees, but so far it has proved impracticable to ensure that all get a period in an established academic department.

The M.R.C.Psych. Examination and Related Examinations

For the guidance of trainees the Court of Electors have issued regulations concerning the Preliminary Test and the Membership Examination. Trainees are advised to obtain from the Royal College of Psychiatrists the latest statements about this examination. Likewise, information about the D.P.M. can be obtained from The Secretary, The Examining Board in England, Examination Hall, 8-11 Queen Square, London, W.C.1. Various University D.P.M.s are still in existence and the respective medical schools provide full information about their requirements and curricula.

Inceptors

Trainees may apply to become Inceptor Members of the Royal College of Psychiatrists. They will receive the British Journal of Psychiatry at reduced rates and be entitled to attend scientific educational meetings organised by the College and by its Regional Divisions in many parts of the country. Inceptors also have the opportunity to play an active part in the life of the College by serving as representatives on various committees.

Approved Hospitals

The clinical psychiatric experience qualifying for entry to the Membership Examination must be obtained in hospitals or units approved by the College for this purpose. A list of such institutions is available from the College and is revised periodically.

Note: Enquiries concerning training to be approved for purposes of taking the examinations should be addressed to the Dean at the College.

Reference

Recommended reference for further information:
Inceptors and Trainees in Psychiatry. Edited by Thomas Bewley (Sub-Dean) for the Education Committee of the Royal College of Psychiatrists, 1976.

ACKNOWLEDGMENT

Special thanks are given to the Royal College of Psychiatrists (London, England) for permission to reprint this material.

Appendix D

Introductory Reading List for Chapter 1*

Section I. Historical Trends in Psychiatry

Major References

Freedman, A. M., et al. Modern Synopsis of the Comprehensive Textbook of Psychiatry. Williams and Wilkins, Baltimore, 1972.

Redlich, F. C., and Freedman, D. X. Theory and Practice of Psychiatry. Basic Books, New York, 1966.

Other References

Alexander, G. F., and Selesnick, S. T. The History of Psychiatry, Harper and Row, New York, 1966.

Ellenberger, H. F. The Discovery of the Unconscious: The History and Evolution of Dynamic Psychiatry. Basic Books, New York, 1970.

Galdston, I. (ed.). Historic Derivations of Modern Psychiatry. McGraw-Hill, New York, 1967.

Zilboorg, G. A. A History of Medical Psychology, W. W. Norton, New York, 1941.

Section II. Normality and Normal Psychosexual Development

A. Normality

Major References

Arieti, S. (ed.). American Handbook of Psychiatry. 2nd ed. Basic Books, New York, 1974.

Freedman, A. M., Kaplan, H. I., and Sadock, B. J. (eds.). Comprehensive Textbook in Psychiatry, II. Williams and Wilkins, Baltimore, 1975.

Other References

Beiser, M. "A Psychiatric Follow-up Study of 'Normal' Adults." Am. J. Psychiatry 127 (1971):1464–1472.

Grinker, R. R., et al. "Mentally Healthy 'Young Males (Homoclites)': A Study." Arch. Gen. Psychiatry 6(1972):405–453.

Offer, D., and Sabshin, M. Normality: Theoretical and Clinical Concepts of Mental Health. Basic Books, New York, 1966.

Szaza, T. S. The Myth of Mental Illness: Foundations of a Theory of Personal Conduct. Hoeber-Harper, New York, 1961.

Bardwick, Judith. The Psychology of Women. Harper and Row, New York, 1972.

---

*This list is intended only as a guide to reading and as a supplement to the lists referred to in Appendix B.

Bardwick, Judith (ed.). *Readings on the Psychology of Women*. Harper and Row, New York, 1972.
Maccoby, Elanor E., and Jacklin, Carol N. *The Psychology of Sex Differences*. Stanford University Press, Stanford, 1974.
Money, J., and Ehrhardt, A. A. *Man and Woman, Boy and Girl*. Johns Hopkins University Press, Baltimore, 1972.

B. Normal Psychosexual Development

Major Reference

Freedman, A. M., Kaplan, H. I., and Sadock, B. J. (eds.). *Comprehensive Textbook in Psychiatry*, II. Williams and Wilkins, Baltimore, 1975.

Other References

Erikson, E. H. "The Eight Ages of Man." In: *Childhood and Society*. 2nd ed. Horton, New York, 1963. pp. 247–274.
Freud, S. *Three Contributions to the Theory of Sex*. Translated by A. A. Brill. Nervous and Mental Disease Monograph Series No. 7, 4th ed. Nervous and Mental Disease Publishing Co., New York, 1930.
Kinsey, A. C., Pomeroy, W. B., and Martin, C. E. *Sexual Behavior in the Human Male*. Saunders, Philadelphia, 1948.
Kinsey, A. C., Pomeroy, W. B., and Martin, C. E. *Sexual Behavior in the Human Female*. Saunders, Philadelphia, 1953.
Masters, W. H., and Johnson, V. E. *Human Sexual Response*. Little, Brown, Boston, 1966.
"Normal Adolescence: Its Dynamics and Impact." *Report of the Group for the Advancement of Psychiatry* 6(1968): 755–851.

Section III. Contributions of the Biological Sciences to Psychiatry

A. Core Knowledge in Neuropsychiatry

Major References

Forrest, A. (ed.). *Companion to Psychiatric Studies*. Longman, New York, 1973.
Freedman, A. M., Kaplan, H. I., and Sadock, B. J. (eds.). *Comprehensive Textbook of Psychiatry*, II. Williams and Wilkins, Baltimore, 1975.
Kral, V. A. "Clinical Contributions Towards an Understanding of Memory Function." *Dis. Nerv. Syst.* 31(1970):23–29.
MacLean, P. D. *A Triune Concept of the Brain and Behavior*. University of Toronto Press, Toronto, 1973.
Plum, F., and Posner, J. B. *The Diagnosis of Stupor and Coma*. 2nd ed. F. A. Davis Co., Philadelphia, 1972.
Victor, M., Adams, R. D., and Collins, G. H. *The Wernicke–Korsakoff Syndrome*. F. A. Davis Co., Philadelphia, 1971.

General Reference

Pryse-Phillips, W., Murray, T. J., *Essential Neurology*, Medical Examination Publishing Co., Inc., Garden City, New York, 1978.

B. Core Knowledge in Neuroendocrinology

Major References

Brown, G. M., and Reichlin, S. "Psychologic and Neural Regulation of Growth Hormone Secretion." *Psychosom. Med.* 34(1972):45–61.
Brown, G. Review. *Am. J. Psychiatry*. 1977.

Prakash, G., Ettigi, and Gregory Brown. "Psychoneuroendocrinology of Affective Disorder: An Overview. *Am. J. Psychiatry* **134**.

Rose, R. M. "The Psychologic Effects of Androgens and Estrogens—A Review." In: *Psychiatric Complications of Medical Drugs*. Chapt. 1. R. I. Shader (ed.). Raven Press, New York, 1972. pp. 251–293.

Smith, C. K., *et al.* "Psychiatric Disturbance in Endocrinologic Disease." *Psychosom. Med.* **34**(1972): 69–86.

See also references in III.D and E.

C. Core Knowledge in Neurochemistry and Neurophysiology and the Relationship of These Sciences to Psychiatric Disorders

Major References

Akiskal, H. S., and McKinney, W. T., Jr. "Depressive Disorders: Toward a Unified Hypothesis." *Science* **183**(1973):20–29.

Arieti, S. (ed.). *American Handbook of Psychiatry*. 2nd ed. Basic Books, New York, 1974.

Detre, T. P., and Jarecki, H. G. *Modern Psychiatric Treatment*. Lippincott, Philadelphia, 1971.

Freedman, A. M., Kaplan, H. I., and Sadock, B. J. (eds.). *Comprehensive Textbook of Psychiatry*, II. Williams and Wilkins, Baltimore, 1975.

Mendels, J. *Biological Psychiatry*. Wiley, New York, 1973.

Smythies, J. R., Coppen, A., and Kreitman, N. *Biological Psychiatry: A Review of Recent Advances*. Heinemann Medical Books, London, 1968.

Snyder, S. H., Banerjee, S. P., Yamamura, H. I., and Greenburg, D. "Drugs, Neurotransmitters, and Schizophrenia." *Science* **184**(1974):1243–1253.

Whybrow, P., and Parlatore, A. "Melancholia: A Model in Madness; A Discussion of Recent Psychobiologic Research into Depressive Illness." *Psychiatry Med.* **4**(1973):351–378.

Other References

Arthur, R. J. "Social Psychiatry: An Overview." *Am. J. Psychiatry* **130**(1973):841–849.

Handler, P. (ed.). *Biology and the Future of Man*. Oxford University Press, New York, 1970.

Klein, D. F., and Davis, J. M. *Diagnosis and Drug Treatment of Psychiatric Disorders*. Williams and Wilkins, Baltimore, 1969.

Maller, O. "The Sociology of Psychiatry." *Confin. Psychiatry.* **9**(1966):129–142.

Pines, M. *The Brain Changers: Scientists and the New Mind Control*. Harcourt Brace Jovanovich, New York, 1973.

Rark, L. C., and Imboden, J. B. "Clinical and Heuristic Value of Clinical Drug Research." *J. Nerv. Ment. Dis.* **151**(1970):322–340.

Rose, S. *The Conscious Brain*. Weidenfeld and Nicolson, London, 1973.

Semrad, E. V. "On the Need for Specificity in the Description of Clinical Function in Somatic Studies of Psychotic Patients." In: *Conference on the Future of the Brain Sciences*, Academy of Medicine, New York, 1968. Edited by P. Bogoch, Plenum Press, New York, 1969.

Thomas, A., *et al. Temperament and Behavior Disorders in Children*. New York University Press, New York, 1968.

D. Memory

Major References

Frontiers of Psychological Research. Readings from Scientific American. W. H. Freeman, San Francisco, 1966.

Psychobiology: The Biological Basis of Behavior. Readings from Scientific American. W. H. Freeman, San Francisco, 1967.

Victor, M. "The Amnestic Syndrome and Its Anatomical Basis." *Can. Med. Assoc. J.* **100**(1969):1115–1125.

Other References

Haber, R. N. "How We Remember What We See." *Sci. Am.* **222** (May, 1970):104–112.
Laughlin, H. P. *The Neuroses.* Butterworths, London, 1967.
Quarton, G. C., *et al. The Neurosciences.* Rockefeller University Press, New York, 1967.

E. Sleep and Dreams

Major References

Broughton, R. "A Proposed Classification of Sleep Disorders." In: *Sleep Research.* Chase, M. H., Stern, W. C., and Walters, P. L. (eds.). UCLA Brain Information Service, Brain Research Institute, Los Angeles, 1972. p. 146.
Broughton, R. J. "Sleep Disorders: Disorders of Arousal?" *Science* **159**(1968):1070–1078.
Dement, W. C., and Guilleminault, C. "Sleep Disorders: The State of the Art." *Hosp. Prac.* S(Nov. 1973):57–71.
Lowy, F. H. "Recent Sleep and Dream Research: Clinical Implications." *Can. Med. Assoc. J.* **102** (1970):1069–1077.
Usdin, G. *Sleep Research and Clinical Practice.* Brunner/Mazel, New York, 1973.

Other References

Aserinsky, E., and Kleitman, N. "Regularly Occurring Periods of Eye Motility and Concomitant Phenomena during Sleep." *Science* **118**(1953):273–274.
Luce, G. G. *Biological Rhythms in Psychiatry and Medicine.* Public Health Service Publication No. 2088, National Institute of Mental Health, Chevy Chase, Maryland, 1970.

Section IV. Contributions of the Psychological Sciences to Psychiatry

General References for All Topics

Freedman, A. N., Kaplan, H. I., and Sadock, B. J. (eds.). *Comprehensive Textbook of Psychiatry*, II. Williams & Wilkins, Baltimore, 1975.
Berelson, B., and Steiner, G. A. *Human Behavior: An Inventory of Scientific Findings.* Harcourt, Brace & World, New York, 1964.
Frontiers of Psychological Research: Readings from Scientific American. W. H. Freeman, San Francisco, 1966.
Mussen, P., *et al. Psychology: An Introduction.* Heath, Lexington, Massachusetts, 1973.
Psychobiology: The Biological Basis of Behavior. Readings from Scientific American. W. H. Freeman, San Francisco, 1967.

A. Motivation

Major Reference

Murray, E. J. *Motivation and Emotion.* Prentice-Hall, Englewood Cliffs, New Jersey, 1964.

Other References

Korman, A. K. *The Psychology of Motivation.* Prentice-Hall, Englewood Cliffs, New Jersey, 1974.
Weiner, B. *Theories of Motivation: From Mechanism to Cognition.* Rand McNally, Chicago, 1972.

B. Ethology

Major Reference

Freedman, A. M., Kaplan, H. I., and Sadock, B. J. (eds.). *Comprehensive Textbook of Psychiatry*, II. Williams and Wilkins, Baltimore, 1975.

C. Cognition

i. Intelligence

Major References

Baldwin, A. L. *Theories of Child Development*. Chapts. 5–9, Wiley, Chicago, 1967.
Phillips, J. L. *The Origins of Intellect: Piaget's Theory*. W. H. Freeman, San Francisco, 1969.
Tyler, L. E. (ed.). *Intelligence: Some Recurring Issues*. Van Nostrand Reinhold, New York, 1969.

Other References

Furth, H. G. *Piaget and Knowledge: Theoretical Foundations*. Prentice-Hall, Englewood Cliffs, New Jersey, 1969.
Meeker, M. N. *The Structure of Intellect: Its Interpretation and Uses*. Merrill, Columbus, Ohio, 1969.

ii. Language Development

Major Reference

Freedman, A. M., Kaplan, H. E., and Sadock, B. J. (eds.). *Comprehensive Textbook of Psychiatry*, II. Williams and Wilkins, Baltimore, 1975.

Other References

Belugi, U. "Learning the Language." *Psychology Today*, December 1970.
Chase, R. A. "Biological Dimensions of Language and Language Disorders in Children." *Bulletin of the Orton Society*, 1968.
Chomsky, N. *Language and Mind*. Harcourt Brace Jovanovich, New York, 1972.
DeHirsch, K. "A Review of Early Language Development." *Dev. Med. Child. Neurol.* 12(1970):87–97.
Eimas, P., *et al.* "Speech Perception in Infants." *Science* 171(1971):303–306.
Lenneberg, E. (ed.). *New Directions in the Study of Language*. MIT Press, Cambridge, 1964.
Marler, P. "Birdsong and Speech Development: Could There Be Parallels?" *Am. Science* 58(1970): 669–673.
McNeill, D. *The Acquisition of Language: The Study of Developmental Psycholinguistics*. Harper and Row, New York, 1970.
Sinclair-de-Zwart, H. "Developmental Psycholinguistics." In: *Studies in Cognitive Development: Essays in Honor of Jean Piaget*. Elkind, D., and Flavell, J. H. (eds.). Oxford University Press, New York, 1969. pp. 315–336.
Skinner, B. F. *Verbal Behavior*. Appleton-Century-Crofts, New York, 1957. pp. 412–413.

D. Perception

Major References

Freedman, A. M., Kaplan, H. I., and Sadock, B. J. (eds.). *Comprehensive Textbook of Psychiatry*, II. Williams and Wilkins, Baltimore, 1975.
Hochberg, J. E. *Perception*. Prentice-Hall, Englewood Cliffs, New Jersey, 1964.

E. General Systems Theory

Major Reference

Miller, J. G. "Living Systems: Basic Concepts." *Behav. Sci.* 10(1965):193–237.

Other References

Bales, R. F. "The Equilibrium Problem in Small Groups." In: *Working Papers in the Theory of Action*. Parsons, T., Bales, R. F., and Shils, B. A. (eds.). The Free Press, Glencoe, Illinois, 1953. pp. 111–161.
Berkman, R. "Phenomenology and General Systems Theory as Methods in Psychotherapy." *Am. J. Psychother.* 26(1973):633–638.

Hearn, G. "The General Systems Approach to the Understanding of Groups." *Health Educ. Monogr.* 14, 1962.

Holder, H. D. "Mental Health and the Search for New Organizational Strategies. *Arch. Gen. Psychiatry* **20**(1969):709–717.

Howells, J. G. *Theory and Practice of Family Psychiatry.* Brunner/Mazel, New York, 1971.

Hutcheson, B. R., and Krause, E. A. "Systems Analysis and Mental Health Services." *Comm. Ment. Health. J.* **5**(1969):29–45.

Meir, A. Z. "General Systems Theory: Developments and Perspectives for Medicine and Psychiatry." *Arch. Gen. Psychiatry* **21**(1969):302–310.

Thompson, M. "A Systems Approach to Delivery of Mental Health Services in North Halton County, Canada." *J. Am. Acad. Child Psychiatry* **14**(Spring 1975).

Von Bertalanffy, L. "General Systems Theory and Psychiatry." In: *American Handbook of Psychiatry.* S. Arieti (ed.). Basic Books, New York, 1966. Vol. 3, Chapt. 43, pp. 705–721.

F. Communications Theory

Major Reference

Freedman, A. M., Kaplan, H. I., and Sadock, B. J. (eds.). *Comprehensive Textbook of Psychiatry,* II. Williams and Wilkins, Baltimore, 1975.

Section V.   Contributions of the Sociocultural Sciences to Psychiatry

A. Cultural Anthropology

Major References

Bell, N. W., and Vogel, E. F. (eds.). *A Modern Introduction to the Family.* Free Press, New York, 1968.

Murphy, H. B. M. "Social Change and Mental Health." In: *Causes of Mental Disorder: A Review of Epidemiological Knowledge, 1959.* Milbank Memorial Fund, New York, 1961. pp. 280–329.

Wallace, A. F. C. "Anthropology and Psychiatry." In: *Comprehensive Textbook of Psychiatry.* Freedman, A. M., Kaplan, H. I. and Sadock, B. J. (eds.). Williams and Wilkins, Baltimore, 1975. pp. 366–373.

Other References

Heath, D. B. "Sexual Division of Labour and Cross-Cultural Research." *Social Forces* **37**(1958):77–79.

Kardiner, A., and Preble, E. *They Studied Man.* Seeker & Warburg. London, 1961.

LeVine, R. A. *Culture, Behaviour and Personality.* Aldine, Chicago, 1973.

Meadows, D. H., *et al. Limits to Growth: A Report for the Club of Rome's Project on the Predicament of Mankind.* Universe Books, New York, 1972.

Murdock, G. P. *Social Structure.* Free Press, New York, 1965.

Toffler, A. *Future Shock.* Bantam Books, New York, 1971.

B. Sociology, Ecology, and Social Psychiatry

Major References

Koenig, S. *Sociology: An Introduction to the Science of Society.* Barnes & Noble, New York, 1962.

Leighton, D. C., and Leighton, A. H. "Mental Health and Social Factors." In: *Comprehensive Textbook of Psychiatry.* Freedman, A. M., and Kaplan, H. I. (eds.). Williams and Wilkins, Baltimore, 1967. pp. 1520–1533.

Report of the Royal Commission on the Status of Women in Canada, Information Canada, Ottawa, 1970.

Huber, Joan (ed.). *Changing Women in a Changing Society,* University of Chicago Press, Chicago, 1973.

Lewis, O. "The Culture of Poverty." *Sci. Am.* **215**(Oct. 1966):19–25.

Ransom, A. *Introduction to Social Psychiatry.* Penguin Books, London.

Silverman, I. "Sociology and Psychiatry." In: *Comprehensive Textbook of Psychiatry*, II. Freedman, A. M., Kaplan, H. I., and Sadock, B. J. (eds.). Williams and Wilkins, Baltimore, 1975. pp. 373–382.

Other References

Caudill, W. *The Psychiatric Hospital as a Small Society.* Harvard University Press, Cambridge, 1958.

Cummings, E., and Cummings, J. *Closed Ranks: An Experiment in Mental Health Education.* Harvard University Press, Cambridge, 1957.

Faris, R. E., and Drenham, H. W. *Mental Disorders in Urban Areas.* University of Chicago Press, Chicago, 1965.

Goffman, E. *Asylums: Essays on the Social Situation of Mental Patients and Other Inmates.* Doubleday, New York, 1961.

Goldhamer, H., and Marshall, A. *Psychosis and Civilization.* Free Press, New York, 1953.

Hollingshead, A. B., and Redlich, F. C. *Social Class and Mental Illness: A Community Study.* Wiley, New York, 1958.

Kesey, K. *One Flew Over the Cuckoo's Nest.* Viking Press, New York, 1962.

Madge, J. H. *The Origins of Scientific Sociology.* Free Press, New York, 1962.

Prince, R. H. "Psychotherapy and the Chronically Poor." In: *Culture Change, Mental Health and Poverty.* J. C. Finne (ed.). University of Kentucky Press, Lexington, 1969. pp. 20–41.

C. Transcultural Psychiatry

Major References

Draguns, J. G. "Comparisons of Psychopathology Across Cultures: Issues, Findings, Directions." *J. Cross-Cultural Psychol.* **4**(1973):10–47.

Leighton, A. H., *et al.* "Therapeutic Process in Cross-Cultural Perspective." *Am. J. Psychiatry* **124** (1968):56–69.

Murphy, H. B. M. "Current Trends in Transcultural Psychiatry." *Proc. R. Soc. Med.* **66**(1973):711–716.

Watts, A. W. *Psychotherapy, East and West.* Ballantine Books, New York, 1969.

Wittkower, E. D., and Dubreuil, G. "Reflections on the Interface between Psychiatry and Anthropology." In: *The Interface between Psychiatry and Anthropology.* I. Galdston (ed.). Brunner/Mazel, New York, 1971. pp. 1–27.

Other References

Kiev, A. *Magic, Faith and Healing.* Free Press, New York, 1974.

La Barre, W. "The Influence of Freud on Anthropology." *Am. Image* **15**(1958):275–328.

Murphy, H. B. M. "Cultural Factors in the Genesis of Schizophrenia." In: *The Transmission of Schizophrenia.* D. Rosenthal and S. S. Kety (eds.). Pergamon Press, Oxford, 1968, pp. 137–153. [Also *J. Psychiat. Res.* **6**(1968) Suppl. 1.]

Yap, P. M. "The Culture-Bound Reactive Syndromes." In: *Mental Health Research in Asia and the Pacific.* W. Caudell and T. Y. Lin (eds.). University of Hawaii Press, Honolulu, 1969. pp. 33–53.

Section VI.   Child and Adolescent Psychiatry

A. Child Psychiatry

i. Child Development

Major References

Baldwin, A. L. *Theories of Child Development.* Wiley, New York, 1967.

Birch, H., Thomas, A., and Chess, S. "The Origin of Personality." *Sci. Am.* **223**:102–109, 1970.

Bowlby, J. "Grief and Mourning in Infancy and Early Childhood." *Psychoanal. Study Child.* **15**:9, 1960.

Eisenberg, L. "Child Psychiatry: The Past Quarter Century." *Am. J. Orthopsychiatry* **39**:389, 1969.
Erikson, E. *Childhood and Society.* Chapt. 7. W. W. Norton & Co., New York, 1963.
Fraiberg, S. H. *The Magic Years.* Scribners, New York, 1959.
Freud, A. *Psycho-Analytical Treatment of Children.* International University Press, New York, 1965.
Ginsberg, H., and Opper, S. *Piaget's Theory of Intellectual Development: An Introduction.* Prentice-Hall, Englewood Cliffs, New Jersey, 1969.
Rutter, M., *et al.* "A New Psychiatric Study in Childhood." *Clin. Dev. Med.* **35/36,** 1970.
Rutter, M. *Maternal Deprivation Reassessed.* Penguin Books, New York, 1972.
Spitz, R. A. "Anaclitic Depression." *Psychoanal. Study Child.* **2**:313–342, 1946.

ii. Syndromes in Child Psychiatry

Major References

Alderton, H. R. "A Review of Schizophrenia in Childhood." *Can. Psychiatr. Assoc. J.* **11**:276, 1966.
Bender, L. "The Nature of Childhood Psychosis." In: *Modern Perspectives of International Child Psychiatry.* John G. Howells (ed.). Chapt. 23. Oliver and Boyd, Edinburgh, 1969.
Hoag, N., *et al.* "The Encopretic Child and His Family." *J. Child Psychiatry* **10**:242, 1971.
Johnson, A. M., and Szurek, S. A. "The Genesis of Antisocial Acting Out in Children and Adults." *Psychoanal. Q.* **21**:323–343, 1952.
Quay, H. C., and Werry, J. S. *Psychopathological Disorders of Childhood.* Wiley, New York, 1972.
Rae-Grant, Q., and Levine, S. V., "School Phobia." *Mod. Med.* **24**:21, 1969.
Robins, L. N., *Deviant Children Grown Up.* Williams and Wilkins, Baltimore, 1966.
Rutter, M. "Concepts of Autism: A Review of Research." *J. Child Psychol.* **9**:1–25, 1968.
Rutter, M. L. "Relationships between Child and Adult Psychiatric Disorders." *Acta Psychiatr. Scand.* **48**:3–21, 1972.
Thompson, L. J. "Learning Disabilities: An Overview." *Am. J. Psychiatry* **130**:393–399, 1973.
Toolan, J. H. "Depression in Children and Adolescents." *Am. J. Orthopsychiatry* **32**:404, 1962.

iii. Treatment in Child Psychiatry

Major References

Berlin, I. N. "Learning Mental Health Consultation, History and Problems." *Ment. Hyg.* **48**:257–266, 1964.
Caplan, G. "Types of Mental Health Consultation." *Am. J. Orthopsychiatry* **33**:470, 1963.
Caplan, G., and Bruenbaum, H. "Perspective on Primary Prevention: A Review." *Arch. Gen. Psychiatry* **17**:331, 1967.
Fish, B. "Drug Use in Psychiatric Disorders of Children." *Am. J. Psychiatry* **124**:8, 641–650, 1968.
Lester, E. P. "Brief Psychotherapies in Child Psychiatry." *Can. Psychiatr. Assoc. J.* **13**:301, 1968.
Moustakas, C. E. *Psychotherapy with Children.* Harper and Row, New York, 1959. Ballantine Paperback, New York, 1973.

iv. Adolescence and Its Problems

Major References

Anthony, E. J. "Clinical Evaluation of Children with Psychotic Parents." *Am. J. Psychiatry* **126**:177, 1969.
Anthony, E. J. "Two Contrasting Types of Adolescent Depression and Their Treatment." *Am. Psychoanal. Assoc. J.* **18**:841, 1970.
Blos, P. Chapt. 3, "Phases of Adolescence"; Chapt. 5, "The Ego in Adolescence." In: *On Adolescence.* Free Press: Dist. by Macmillan Co., New York, 1962.
Golembek, H. "The Therapeutic Contact with Adolescents." *Can. Psychiatr. Assoc. J.* **14**:497, 1969.

Masterson, J. *Treatment of the Borderline Adolescent: A Developmental Approach*. Wiley, New York, 1972.
Weiner, I. B. *Psychological Disturbance in Adolescence*. Wiley, New York, 1970.

v. Psychiatric Problems of the Child and Family

Major References

Bowen, M. "The Use of Family Theory in Clinical Practice." *Compr. Psychiatry* 7:345–374, 1966.
Fine, S. "Troubled Families: Parameters for Diagnosis and Strategies for Change." *Compr. Psychiatry* 15:73–77, 1974.
Foley, V. D. *An Introduction to Family Therapy*. New York, Grune & Stratton, 1974.
Haley, J. "Approaches to Family Therapy." *Int. J. Psychiatry* 9:233–242, 1970.
Lidz, T., Fleck, S., and Cornelison, R. "Schizophrenia and the Family." In: *Family Studies and a Theory of Schizophrenia*. International Universities Press, New York, 1965. Chapter 20.
Minuchin, S. *Families and Family Therapy*. Harvard University Press, Cambridge, 1974.

B. Mental Retardation

Major References

Group for the Advancement of Psychiatry. *Mental Retardation: A Family Crisis—The Therapeutic Role of the Physician*. Report No. 56. December, 1963.
Group for the Advancement of Psychiatry. *Mild Mental Retardation: A Growing Challenge to the Physician*. Report No. 66, September, 1967.
Menolascino, F. J. *Psychiatric Approaches to Mental Retardation*. Basic Books, New York–London, 1970.

C. Genetics

Major Reference

Slater, E., and Cowie, V. *Genetics of Mental Disorder*. Oxford University Press, London–Oxford, 1971.

General Reference for All Areas

Steinhauer, P. D., and Rae-Grant, Q. (eds.). *Psychological Problems for the Child and His Family*, Macmillan of Canada, 1977.

Section VII. Theories of Personality and Psychopathology

Major References

Aufreiter, J. "The Dilemma with Aggression: Primary Need or Consequence of Frustration." *Can. Psychiatr. Assoc. J.* 14:493–496, 1969.
Axline, V. M. *Dibs: In Search of Self*. Ballantine Books, New York, 1969.
Bowlby, J. *Attachment and Loss*. Basic Books, New York, 1969.
Bowlby, J. "The Nature of the Child's Tie to His Mother." *Int. J. Analysis* 38:350, 1958.
Fraiberg, S. H. *The Magic Years*. Scribner, New York, 1959.
Freedman, A. M., Kaplan, H. I., and Sadock, B. J. (eds.). *Comprehensive Textbook of Psychiatry*, II, Williams and Wilkins, Baltimore, 1975.
Freud, A. *The Ego and Mechanisms of Defense*. Hogarth Press, London, 1966.
Hall, C. S., and Lindzey, G. *Theories of Personality*. Chapts. 3 and 4. Wiley, New York, 1965.
Harlow, H. F., and Novak, M. A. "Psychopathological Perspectives." *Perspect. Biol. Med.* 16:461–478, 1973.
Spitz, R. A. *The First Year of Life*. International Universities Press, New York, 1965.
Storr, A. *Human Aggression*. Penguin Books, Harmondsworth, England, 1968.

Other References

Bettelheim, B. *Children of the Dream*. Macmillan, New York, 1969.

Brenner, C. *An Elementary Textbook of Psychoanalysis*. International Universities Press, New York, 1973.

Brown, J. A. C. *Freud and the Post-Freudians*. Penguin Books, New York, 1964.

Erikson, E. *Childhood and Society*. Norton, New York, 1950.

Erikson, E. "Identity and the Life Cycle." *Psychol. Issues.* **1**, 1959.

Freud, S. *A General Introduction to Psychoanalysis*. Liveright, New York, 1974.

Freud, S. "Introductory Lectures on Psychoanalysis." In: *The Standard Edition of the Complete Psychological Works of Sigmund Freud*. J. Strachey (ed.). Hogarth Press, London, 1966. Volumes XV and XVI.

Freud, S. *New Introductory Lectures on Psychoanalysis*. Hogarth Press, London, 1965.

Fromm, E. *The Sane Society*. Holt, Rinehart & Winston, New York, 1955.

Harlow, H. F. "Social Deprivation in Monkeys." *Sci. Am.* **207**:136–146, Nov. 1962.

Horney, K. *Our Inner Conflicts*. Norton, New York, 1945.

Maker, B. A. *Principles of Psychopathology*. McGraw-Hill, New York, 1966. Chapts. 4, 12–15.

Munro, R. L. *Schools of Psychoanalytic Thought*. Dryden Press, New York, 1955.

The Neurosciences—Second Study Program. F. O. Schmitt (ed.). Rockefeller University Press, New York, 1970. Chapts. 1–4, 29–35.

Psychobiology: The Biological Basis of Behavior. Readings from Scientific American. W. H. Freeman, San Francisco, 1966.

Rutter, M. "Maternal Deprivation Reconsidered." *J. Psychosom. Res.* **16**:241–250, 1972.

Storr, A. *Human Aggression*. Penguin Books, New York, 1968.

Sullivan, H. S. *The Interpersonal Theory of Psychiatry*. Norton, New York, 1953.

Section VIII. Psychiatric Assessment

A. The Interview

Major References

Freedman, A. M., Kaplan, H. I., and Sadock, B. J. (eds.). *Comprehensive Textbook of Psychiatry*, II. Williams and Wilkins, Baltimore, 1975.

Kreihman, N. "The Reliability of Psychiatric Diagnosis." *J. Ment. Sci.* **107**:876, Sept. 1961.

MacKinnon, R. A., and Michels, R. *The Psychiatric Interview in Clinical Practice*. Saunders, Philadelphia, 1971.

Sutherland, J. D. "A Psychodynamic Approach to the Understanding of the Person. In: *Companion to Psychiatric Studies*, Vol. I. A. Forrest (ed.). Longman, New York, 1973. Chapt. 10.

Walton, H., and Littman, S. "Interview Methods." In: *Companion to Psychiatric Studies*, Vol. I. A. Forrest (ed.). Longman, New York, 1973. Chapt. 11.

B. Assessment in Psychiatry

Major References

Freedman, A. M., Kaplan, H. I., and Sadock, B. J. (eds.). *Comprehensive Textbook of Psychiatry*, II. Williams and Wilkins, Baltimore, 1975.

Weitzel, W. D., *et al.* "Towards a More Efficient Mental Status Examination—Free Form or Operationally Defined." *Arch. Gen. Psychiatry* **28**:215–218, 1973.

C. Nosology

Major References

Diagnostic Statistics Manuals I and *II* (DSM).

Hampel, C. G. "Some Problems of Taxonomy." In: *Work Conference on Problems in Field Studies in the Mental Disorders*. J. Zukin (ed.). Grune & Stratton, New York, 1959.

Psychopathology: Contributions from the Social, Behavioral and Biological Sciences. M. Hammer et al. (eds.). New York, Wiley, 1973. Chapts. 21, 22.

U.S. Department of Health, Education and Welfare. National Center for Health Statistics. *International Classification of Diseases.* 8th Rev. Washington, D.C., 1969, 2 volumes.

Zilboorg, G. *A History of Medical Psychology.* Norton, New York, 1941. Chapt. 10.

Section IX. Psychiatric Emergencies and Reactive Disorders

A. Crisis Theory

Major References

Caplan, G. *Principles of Preventive Psychiatry.* Basic Books, New York, 1964.

Caplan, G., and Gruenbaum, H. "Perspectives on Primary Prevention." *Arch. Gen. Psychiatry* 17:331–346, 1967.

Langsley, D. G. "Crisis of Intervention." *Am. J. Psychiatry* 129:734–736, 1972.

Lindemann, E. "Symptomatology and Management of Acute Grief." *Am. J. Psychiatry* 101:141–148, 1944.

B. Psychiatric Emergencies

Major Reference

Morrice, J. K. W. "Emergency Psychiatry." *Br. J. Psychiatry* 114:485–491, 1968.

Other References

Kellner, R. "Outlines of the Management of Common Psychiatric Crises and Emergencies in the Community." *Psychosom. Med.* 12:191–199, 1971.

Nigro, S. A. "A Psychiatrist's Experiences in General Practice in a Hospital Emergency Room." *J. Am. Med. Assoc.* 214:1957–1960, 1970.

Whiteley, J. S., and Denison, D. M. "The Psychiatric Casualty." *Br. J. Psychiatry* 109:488–490, 1963.

C. Suicide

Major References

Kessel, N. "Self-Poisoning. Part I." *Br. Med. J.* 2:1265–1270, 1965.

Kreitman, N., et al. "Parasuicide." *Br. J. Psychiatry* 116:460–461, 1970.

McCarthy, P. D., and Walsh, D. "Suicide in Dublin." *Br. Med. J.* 1:1393–1396, 1966.

Other References

Dorpat, T. L., and Ripley, H. S. "The Relationship between Attempted Suicide and Committed Suicide." *Compr. Psychiatry* 8:74–79, 1967.

Dublin, L. I. *Suicide: A Sociological and Statistical Study.* Ronald Press, New York, 1963.

Durkheim, E. *Suicide.* Free Press, New York, 1951.

Greer, S., and Bagley, C. "Effect of Psychiatric Intervention in Attempted Suicide: A Controlled Study." *Br. Med. J.* 1:310–312, 1971.

Kessel, N., and McCulloch, J. W. "Repeated Acts of Self-Poisoning and Self-Injury." *Proc. R. Soc. Med.* 59:89–92, 1966.

Philip, A. E., and McCulloch, J. W. "Use of Social Indices in Psychiatric Epidemiology." *Br. J. Prev. Soc. Med.* 20:122–126, 1966.

Rosen, D. H. "The Serious Suicide Attempt: Epidemiological and Follow-up Study of 886 Patients." *Am. J. Psychiatry* 127:765–770, 1970.

Stengel, E., and Cook, N. G. *Attempted Suicide.* Oxford University Press, New York, 1958.

D. Transient Situational Disturbances

i. Stress Reaction

Major Reference

Tyhurst, J. S. "Individual Reactions to Community Disaster." *Am. J. Psychiatry* **107**:764–769, 1951.

ii. Acute Grief Reaction

Major References

Parkes, C. M. "Anticipatory Grief and Widowhood." *Br. J. Psychiatry* **122**:615, May 1973.
Parkes, C. M. "Bereavement and Mental Illness. 1. A Clinical Study of the Grief of Bereaved Psychiatric Patients." *Br. J. Med. Psychol.* **38**:1–12, March 1965.
Parkes, C. M. "Bereavement and Mental Illness. 2. A Classification of Bereavement Reactions." *Br. J. Med. Psychol.* **38**:13–26, March 1965.
Lindemann, E. "Symptomatology and Management of Acute Grief." *Am. J. Psychiatry* **101**:141–148, 1944.

iii. Combat Neuroses

Major References

Caldwell, J. M. "Military Psychiatry." In: *Comprehensive Textbook of Psychiatry*. A. M. Freedman and H. I. Kaplan (eds.). Williams and Wilkins, Baltimore, 1967. Chapt. 49, pp. 1605–1612.
Sargant, W. *Battle for the Mind*. Harper & Row, New York, 1971.

iv. Acute Culture-Bound Reactions

Major References

Lehmann, H. "Unusual Psychiatric Disorders and Atypical Psychoses." In: *Comprehensive Textbook of Psychiatry*. A. M. Freedman and H. I. Kaplan (eds.). Williams and Wilkins, Baltimore, 1967. Chapt. 32, pp. 1150–1161.
Yap, P. M. "Koro—A Culture-Bound Depersonalization Syndrome." *Br. J. Psychiatry* **111**:43–50, 1965.

Section X.   Psyche and Soma and Liaison Psychiatry

Major References

Bain, S. T., and Spaulding, W. B. "The Importance of Coding Presenting Symptoms." *Can. Med. Assoc. J.* **97**:953–959, 1967.
Freedman, A. M., Kaplan, H. I., and Sadock, B. J. (eds.). *Comprehensive Textbook of Psychiatry*, II. Williams and Wilkins, Baltimore, 1975.
Lipowski, Z. J. "Psychosomatic Medicine in the Seventies: An Overview." *Am. J. Psychiatry* **134**:3, 1977.
Rahe, R. H., *et al.* "Social Stress and Illness Onset." *J. Psychosom. Res.* **8**:35–44, 1964.
Shapiro, A. P., *et al. Psychosomatic Classics: Selected Papers from Psychosomatic Medicine*. Karger, Basel, 1971.

Other References

Chodoff, P., and Lyons, H. "Hysteria of the Hysterical Personality and Hysterical Conversion." *Am. J. Psychiatry* Vol. II **47**:34/740, 1958.
Hinkle, L. W., and Wolff, H. G. "A Brief for the Investigation of Human Ecology." *Clin. Res.* **5**:127–128, 1957.
Hinkle, L. W., and Wolff, H. G. "Ecologic Investigations of the Relationship between Illness, Life Experiences, and the Social Environment." *Ann. Intern. Med.* **49**:1373–1388, 1958.

Holmes, T. H., and Rahe, R. H. "The Social Readjustment Rating Scale." *J. Psychosom. Res.* **11**:213–218, 1967.

Merskey, H. "Psychological Aspects of Pain," *Postgrad. Med. J.* **44**:297–306, 1968.

Roghmann, K. J., and Haggerty, R. J. "Daily Stress, Illness and Use of Health Services in Young Families." *Pediatr. Res.* **7**:520–526, 1973.

Thurlow, H. J. "General Susceptibility to Illness: A Selective Review." *Can. Med. Assoc. J.* **97**:1397–1404, 1967.

Section XI.   The Neuroses, Personality Disorders, Addictions, and Sexual Disorders

Major References

Freedman, A. M., Kaplan, H. I., and Sadock, B. J. (eds.). *"Comprehensive Textbook of Psychiatry,* II. Williams and Wilkins, Baltimore, 1975.

MacKibben, R., and Michels, R. *Psychiatric Interview in Clinical Practice.* Saunders, Philadelphia, 1971.

Slater, E., and Roth, M. (eds.) *Clinical Psychiatry.* 3rd ed. Bailliert, Tindall & Cassell, London, 1969.

Other Reference

Laughlin, H. P. *The Neuroses in Clinical Practice.* Saunders, Philadelphia, 1956.

Section XII.   The "Functional" Psychoses

General References for All Topics

Freedman, A. M., Kaplan, H. I., and Sadock, B. J. (eds.). *Comprehensive Textbook of Psychiatry,* II. Williams and Wilkins, Baltimore, 1975.

International Classification of Diseases, 8th rev. Vol. 2. U.S. Department of Health, Education and Welfare, Superintendent of Documents, U.S. Government Printing Office, Washington, D.C.

Manual for the Classification of Psychiatric Diagnosis, based on *International Classification of Diseases* (ICDA-8). Dominion Bureau of Statistics, Health and Welfare Division, Mental Health Section, The Queen's Printer, Ottawa, 1969.

A. The Schizophrenic Disorders

Arieti, S. "Schizophrenia: The Manifest Symptomatology, the Psychodynamics and Formal Mechanisms." In: *American Handbook of Psychiatry.* S. Arieti (ed.). Vol. 1, Chapt. 23. Basic Books, New York, 1959. pp. 455–484.

Ban, T. A. *Schizophrenia: A Psychological Approach.* Charles C. Thomas, Springfield, Illinois, 1972.

Bleuler, E. *Dementia Praecox: Or the Group of Schizophrenias.* Translated by J. Zinkin. International Universities Press, New York, 1969.

Cameron, N. "One Paranoid Pseudo-Community Revised." *Am. J. Sociol.* **44**:152, 1963.

Coppen, A., and Walk, A. (eds.). *Recent Developments in Schizophrenia.* Headley, Ashford, 1967.

Davidson, K., and Bagley, C. R. "Schizophrenia-Like Psychoses Associated with Organic Disorders of the Central Nervous System: A Review of the Literature." In: *Current Problems in Neuropsychiatry.* R. N. Herrinton (ed.). Part 2. Royal Medico-Psychological Association, Ashford, Kent, 1969.

Fish, F. J. *Schizophrenia.* Wright, Bristol, 1962.

Kay, D. W. K. "Schizophrenia and Schizophrenia-Like States in the Elderly." *Br. J. Hosp. Med.* **8**: 369–376, 1972.

Kendall, R. E. "Schizophrenia: The Remedy for Diagnostic Confusion." *Br. J. Hosp. Med.* **8**:383–390, 1972.

Ketty, S. S. "Biochemical Theories of Schizophrenia." *Int. J. Psychiatry* **1**:409–446, 1965.

May, P. R., *et al. Treatment of Schizophrenia: A Comparative Study of Five Treatment Methods.* Aronson, New York, 1968.

Mellor, C. S. "First Rank Symptoms of Schizophrenia." *Br. J. Psychiatry* **117**: 15–23, 1970.
Payne, R. W. "Cognitive Abnormalities." In: *Handbook of Abnormal Psychology*. H. J. Eysenck (ed.). Knapp, San Diego, 1973.
Rosenthal, D., and Ketty, S. S. (eds.). *The Transmission of Schizophrenia*. Pergamon Press, Oxford, 1968.
Slater, E., and Roth, M. (eds.). "Schizophrenia." In: *Clinical Psychiatry*. 3rd ed. Bailliere, Tindall & Cassell, London, 1969. Chapt. 5.
Wing, J. K. "Epidemiology of Schizophrenia." *Br. J. Hosp. Med.* **8**:364–368, 1972.

B. Paranoid Disorders

Erikson, E. H. "Basic Trust Deficiency." In: *Childhood and Society*. W. W. Norton, New York, 1950. Chapt. 7.
Fish, F. J. "Paranoid States." In: *Schizophrenia*. Wright, Bristol, 1962. pp. 77–101.
Jaspers, K. *General Psychopathology*. 7th ed. Manchester University Press, Manchester, 1963.
Kraepelin, E. *Manic-Depressive Insanity and Paranoia*. Livingstone, Edinburgh, 1921.
Verbeek, E. "De la Paranoia." *Psychiatr. Neurol.* **137**:257–281, 1959.

C. Affective Disorders—Psychotic

Akiskol, H. S., and McKinney, W. T. "Overview of Recent Research in Depression." *Arch. Gen. Psychiatry* **32**, March, 1975.
Davies, B., *et al. Depressive Illness: Some Research Studies*. Charles C. Thomas, Springfield, Illinois, 1972.
Kline, N. S. *Depression: Its Diagnosis and Treatment*. Brunner/Mazel, New York, 1969.
Jacobsen, E. *Depression*. International Universities Press, New York, 1971.
Mendels, J. *Concepts of Depression*. Wiley, New York, 1970.

D. "Borderline" States

Deutsch, M. "Some Forms of Emotional Disturbances and Their Relationship to Schizophrenia." *Psychoanalysis* **11**:103–321, 1942.
Grinker, R. R., *et al. The Borderline Syndrome*. Basic Books, New York, 1968.
Hoch, P., and Polatin, P. "Pseudoneurotic Forms of Schizophrenia." *Psychiatr. Q.* **23**:248–276, 1949.
Schmideberg, M. *The Borderline Syndromes*. Basic Books, New York, 1973.

E. Brief Reactive Psychoses

No specific references recommended.

F. Atypical "Psychoses"

Cerrolaza, M., and Cleghorn, R. A. "A Search for Certainty in This Ambiguous Borderland." *Can. Psychiatr. Assoc. J.* **16**:507–514, 1971.
Cohen, S. M., *et al.* The Relationship of Schizo-Affective Psychosis and Schizophrenia. *Arch. Gen. Psychiatry* **26**:539–546, 1972.
Fish, F. J. *Schizophrenia*. Wright, Bristol, 1962. pp. 58–64, 92–104.
Hoch, P., and Polatin, P. "Pseudoneurotic Forms of Schizophrenia." *Psychiatr. Q.* **23**:248–276, 1949.
Leonhard, K. "Cycloid Psychoses: Endogenous Psychoses Which Are Neither Schizophrenia nor Manic-Depressive." *J. Ment. Sci.* **107**:633–648, 1961.

G. Other Psychoses

Brew, M. F., and Seidenberg, R. "Psychotic Reactions Associated with Pregnancy and Childbirth." *J. Nerv. Ment. Dis.* **111**:408–423, 1950.

Brill, A. A. "Piblokoto or Hysteria among Peary's Eskimos." *J. Nerv. Ment. Dist.* **40**:514–520, 1913.

Dalton, K. "Prospective Study into Puerperal Depression." *Br. J. Psychiatry* **118**:689–692, 1971.

Enoch, M. D., *et al. Some Uncommon Psychiatric Syndromes.* Wright, Bristol, 1967.

Granville-Grossman, K. L. (ed.). *Recent Advances in Clinical Psychiatry.* Churchill Livingstone, Edinburgh, 1971, pp. 300–310.

Hemphill, R. E. "Incidence and Nature of Puerperal Psychiatric Illness." *Br. Med. J.* **2**:1232–1235, 1952.

Kretschmer, E. *A Textbook of Medical Psychology.* 2nd English ed. Hogarth, London, 1952.

Nagache, E. *La Jalousie Amoureuse.* Presses Universitaires de France, Paris, 1947.

Nielson, A., and Almgren, P. E. "Paranatal Emotional Adjustment." *Acta. Psychiatr. Scand.*, Suppl. 220, pp. 1–137, 1970.

Tetlow, C. "Psychoses of Childbearing." *J. Ment. Sci.* **101**:629–639, 1955.

Yap, P. M. "Mental Diseases Peculiar to Certain Cultures: A Survey of Comparative Psychiatry." *J. Ment. Sci.* **97**:313–327, 1951.

Section XIII. The Organic Mental Disorders

Major References

Davidson, K. and Bagley, C. R. "Schizophrenia-Like Psychoses Associated with Organic Disorders of the Central Nervous System: A Review of the Literature." In: *Current Problems in Neuropsychiatry.* R. N. Herrington (ed.). *Br. J. Psychiatry* Special Publication No. 4, pp. 113–184, 1969.

Freedman, A. M., Kaplan, H. I., and Sadock, B. J. (eds.). *Comprehensive Textbook of Psychiatry,* II. Williams and Wilkins, Baltimore, 1975.

Herrington, R. N. "The Personality in Temporal Lobe Epilepsy." In: *Current Problems in Neuropsychiatry.* R. N. Herrington (ed.). *Br. J. Psychiatry* Special Publication No. 4, pp. 70–76, 1969.

Lishman, W. A. "The Psychiatric Sequelae of Head Injury: A Review." *Psychol. Med.* **3**:304–318, 1973.

Piercy, M. "The Effects of Cerebral Lesions on Intellectual Function: A Review of Current Research Trends." *Br. J. Psychiatry* **110**:310–352, 1964.

Sim, M. *et al.* "Cerebral Biopsy in the Investigation of Presenile Dementia. I. Clinical Aspects." *Br. J. Psychiatry* **112**:119–125, 1966.

Slater, E., *et al.* "The Schizophrenia-Like Psychoses of Epilepsy." *Br. J. Psychiatry* **109**:95–150, 1963.

Surridge, D. "An Investigation into Some Psychiatric Aspects of Multiple Sclerosis." *Br. J. Psychiatry* **115**:749–764.

Section XIV. The Organic Therapies

A. Psychopharmacology

Major References

Ban, T. A. *Psychopharmacology.* Krieger, New York, 1969.

Drug Interaction Index. Compiled and edited by B. R. Gant and D. T. Gant, Meditec Publications, Vancouver, B.C., 1973 (new replacement pages mailed to subscribers quarterly).

Evaluations of Drug Interactions. 2nd ed. American Pharmaceutical Association, Washington, D.C., 1976.

Goodman, L. S., and Gilman, A. *Pharmacological Basis of Therapeutics.* 4th ed. Macmillan, New York, 1970.

Hansten, P. D. *Drug Interactions: Clinical Significance of Drug–Drug Interactions and Drug Effects on Clinical Laboratory Results.* Lea and Febiger, Philadelphia, 1973.

Martindale, W. H. *The Extra Pharmacopoeia.* 26th ed. Pharmaceutical Press, London, 1972.

Shepherd, M., *et al. Clinical Psychopharmacology.* Lea and Febiger, Philadelphia, 1968.

B. Convulsive Therapies

Major References

Conference: *Psychobiology of Convulsive Therapy*, Dorado Beach, 1972. M. Fink (ed.). Winston, Washington, 1974.

Kalinowsky, L. B., *et al. Pharmacological, Convulsive and Other Somatic Treatments in Psychiatry.* Grune & Stratton, New York, 1969.

Paterson, A. S. *Electrical and Drug Treatments in Psychiatry.* Elsevier, New York, 1963.

Sargant, W. W., and Slater, E. *Introduction to Physical Methods of Treatment in Psychiatry.* 5th ed. Churchill Livingstone, Edinburgh, 1972.

C. Psychosurgery

Major References

Freedman, A. M., Kaplan, H. I., and Sadock, B. J. (eds.). *Comprehensive Textbook of Psychiatry,* II. Williams and Wilkins, Baltimore, 1975.

Kalinowsky, L. B., *et al. Pharmacological, Convulsive, and Other Somatic Treatments in Psychiatry.* Grune & Stratton, New York, 1969.

Sargant, W. W., and Slater, E. *Introduction to Physical Methods of Treatment in Psychiatry.* 5th ed. Churchill Livingstone, Edinburgh, 1972.

D. Miscellaneous and Little-Used Biological Treatments

Major References

Dally, P. J. *Anorexia Nervosa.* Heinemann, London, 1969.

Kalinowsky, L. B., *et al. Pharmacological, Convulsive, and Other Somatic Treatments in Psychiatry.* Grune & Stratton, New York, 1969.

Sargant, W. W., and Slater, E. *Introduction to Physical Methods of Treatment in Psychiatry.* 5th ed. Churchill Livingstone, Edinburgh, 1972.

Section XV.   Learning Theory and Behavior Modification

Major Reference
Bandura, A. *Principles of Behavior Modification.* Holt, Rinehart & Winston, New York, 1969.

Other References

Annual Review of Behavior Therapy. C. M. Franks and T. Wilson (eds.). Brunner/Mazel, New York, 1973.

Behavior Modification: Principles and Clinical Modification. S. Agras (ed.). Little, Brown, Boston, 1972.

Meyer, V., and Chesser, E. S. *Behavior Therapy in Clinical Psychiatry.* Penguin Books, Harmondsworth, 1970.

Miklaus, W. *Concepts in Learning.* Saunders, Philadelphia, 1974.

Schaefer, H. H., and Martin, P. L. *Behavior Therapy.* McGraw-Hill, New York, 1969.

Wolpe, J. *The Practice of Behavior Therapy.* 1st ed. Pergamon Press, New York, 1969. (2nd ed., 1973.)

Section XVI.   The Psychotherapies

Note: It is suggested that the following list be referred to:

Kendall, R. E., and Smith, A. C. (eds.). Royal College of Psychiatrists, Clinical Tutors Subcommittee, Reading List in Psychiatry. 3d ed. Obtainable from the *British Journal of Psychiatry,* Headley Brothers, Ashford, Kent.

Also:

Broverman, Inge D., *et al.* "Sex Role Stereotypes and Clinical Judgments of Mental Health." *J. Consulting Clin. Psychol.* 34:1–7, 1970.

Chesler, Phyllis. *Women and Madness.* Doubleday, New York, 1970.

Franks, Violet, and Burtle, Vasanti. *Women in Therapy: New Psychotherapies for a Changing Society.* Brunner/Mazel, New York, 1974.

Guerin, Philip J. (ed.). *Family Therapy.* Gardner Press, New York, 1976.

Hadley, S. W., and Strupp, H. "Contemporary Views of Negative Effects in Psychotherapy." *Arch. Gen. Psychiatry* 33(11):1291, 1976.

Saul, Leon J. *Psychodynamically Based Psychotherapy.* Science House, New York, 1972.

Wells, R., Trivelli, N., and Dilkes, T. "The Results of Family Therapy: A Critical Review of the Literature." *Family Process* 11(2):189, 1972.

Yalom, Irvin D. *The Theory and Practice of Group Psychotherapy.* 2nd ed. Basic Books, New York, 1975.

Section XVII. Community and Administrative Psychiatry

Major References

Bailey, R. M. "An Economist's View of the Health Services Industry." In: *Health Care Administration.* S. Levey and N. P. Loomba (eds.). Lippincott, Philadelphia, 1973.

Beckhard, R. "Organizational Issues in the Team Delivery of Comprehensive Health Care." *Milbank Mem. Fund. Q.* 50(Part I):287–316, July, 1972.

Costello, C. G. *Psychology for Psychiatrists.* Pergamon Press, Oxford, 1966.

De Alarcon, R. A. "A Personal Medical Reference Index: How to Approach This Life Long Professional Investment." *Lancet* 1:301–305, 1969.

French, C. W. "Evaluation of a Community Mental Health Service." *Social Work Today* 2:22, 1971.

General Notes on the Preparation of Scientific Papers. 2nd ed. Royal Society, 1965.

Glass, N. J. "Cost Benefit Analysis and Health Services." *Health Trends* 5:1973.

Hill, A. B. "Reflections on the Controlled Trial." *Ann. Rheum. Dis.* 25:107–113, 1966.

Ingham, J. G. "Quantitative Evaluation of Subjective Symptoms." *Proc. R. Soc. Med.* 62:492–494, 1969.

Krietman, N. "The Reliability of Psychiatric Diagnosis." *J. Ment. Sci.* 107:876–886, 1961.

Lionel, N. D. W., and Herxheimer, A. "Assessing Reports of Therapeutic Trials." *Br. Med. J.* 3:637–640, 1970.

Mechanic, D. *Mental Health and Social Policy.* Prentice-Hall, Englewood Cliffs, New Jersey, 1969.

Rubin, I. M., and Beckhard, R. "Factors Influencing the Effectiveness of Health Teams." *Milbank Mem. Fund. Q.* 50(Part I):317–335, July, 1972.

Seder, R. E. "Planning and Politics in the Allocation of Health Resources." *Am. J. Pub. Health* 63:774–777, 1973.

Thompson, M. G. G. "New Perspective for Mental Health Care Delivery Systems." *Can. Psychiatr. Assoc. J.* 18:501–504, 1973.

Thorne, C. *Better Medical Writing.* Pitman Medical and Scientific, London, 1970.

Section XVIII. Geriatric and Forensic Psychiatry

A. Geriatric Psychiatry

Major References

Butler, R. N., and Lewis, M. I. *Aging and Mental Health.* C. V. Mosby, St. Louis, 1973.

Kay, D. W. K., and Walk, A. (eds.). *Recent Developments in Psychogeriatrics: A Symposium.* Headley (for Royal Medico-Psychological Association), Ashford, Kent, 1971.

Slater, E., and Roth, M. *Clinical Psychiatry.* 3rd ed. Bailliere, Tindall & Cassell, London, 1969. Chapt. X.

Weinberg, J. "Geriatric Psychiatry." In: *Comprehensive Textbook of Psychiatry,* II. A. M. Freedman, H. I. Kaplan, and B. J. Sadock (eds.). Williams & Wilkins, Baltimore, 1975.

Other References

Erikson, E. H. "Identity and the Life Cycle." *Psychol. Issues* **1**, Monogr. 1, International Universities Press, New York, 1959.

Kubler-Ross, E. *On Death and Dying.* Macmillan, New York, 1969.

Schoenberg, B., *et al.* (eds.). *Psychosocial Aspects of Terminal Care.* Columbia University Press, New York, 1972.

B. Forensic Psychiatry

Major References

Davidson, H. A. *Forensic Psychiatry.* Ronald Press, New York, 1952.

Freedman, A. M., Kaplan, H. I., and Sadock, B. J. (eds.). *Modern Synopsis of the Comprehensive Textbook of Psychiatry,* II. Williams & Wilkins, Baltimore, 1972.

Henderson, D. K. *Textbook in Psychiatry.* 10th ed. Oxford University Press, London, 1969.

Still, L. *Limits of Sanity.* McClelland & Stewart, Toronto, 1972.

Swadron, B., and Sullivan, D. R. (eds.). *Law and Mental Disorder.* Report of the Committee on Legislation and Psychiatric Disorders. Canadian Mental Health Association, Toronto, 1973.

"U.S. Appeals Court Junks Weirham Rule on Insanity." *Psychiatr. News* **7**:14, July 19, 1972.

Section XIX.   Gender and Psychiatry

Due to the relatively new emphasis being given to gender and psychiatry, standard reference lists and texts do not cover this subject as well as they do most others. For this reason, the following relatively comprehensive reference list is included:

General References for All Topics

Chesler, Phyllis. *Women and Madness.* Doubleday, New York, 1970.

Smith, Dorothy E., and David, Sara J. (eds.). *Women Look at Psychiatry.* Vancouver, Press Gang Publishers, 1975.

Stephenson, P. Susan, and Walker, Gillian A. *Women and the Psychiatric Paradox* (in press).

Weitz, Shirley. *Sex Roles: Biological, Psychological and Social Foundations.* Oxford University Press, New York, 1977.

Major References for Each Topic

A. Emerging Issues in the Psychology of Women and Men

Miller, Jean Baker. *Toward a New Psychology of Women.* Beacon Press, Boston, 1976.

Tooley, Kay M. "'Johnny, I Hardly Knew Ye'; toward Revision of the Theory of Male Psychosexual Development." *Am. J. Orthopsychiatry* **47**:184–195, 1977.

B. Sociocultural Aspects

Beauvoir, Simone de. *The Second Sex.* Knopf, New York, 1953.

Janeway, Elizabeth. *Man's World, Woman's Place: A Study in Social Mythology.* Delta Books, New York, 1971.

C. Special Topics

Seiden, Anne M. "Overview: Research on the Psychology of Women. I. Gender Differences and Sexual and Reproductive Life. II. Women in Families, Work and Psychotherapy." *Am. J. Psychiatry* **133**:995–1007; 1111–1123, 1976.

D. Psychotherapy

Broverman, Inge K., *et al.* "Sex Role Stereotypes and Clinical Judgements of Mental Health." *J. Consulting Clin. Psychol.* **34**:1–7, 1970.

Franks, Violet, and Burtle, Vasanti. *Women in Therapy, New Psychotherapies for a Changing Society*. Brunner/Mazel, New York, 1974.

Other References

(These are references that are not cited in the index of Freedman, A. M., Kaplan, H. I., and Sadock, B. J. *Comprehensive Textbook of Psychiatry*. 2nd ed. Williams and Wilkins, Baltimore, 1975.)

Adler, F. *Sisters in Crime: The Rise of the New Female Criminal*. McGraw-Hill, New York, 1975.

Arms, S., *The Immaculate Deception: A New Look at Women and Childbirth in America*. Houghton Mifflin, Boston, 1975.

Bart, P. "Depression in Middle Aged Women." In: Gornick, V., and Moran, B. (eds.). *Women in Sexist Society*. Basic Books, New York, 1971.

Bernard, J. *The Future of Motherhood*. Penguin Books, New York, 1974.

Bernardez-Bonesatti, T. "Women and Anger: Conflicts with Aggression in Contemporary Women." Paper presented at the American Psychiatric Association annual meeting, Toronto, May 4, 1977.

Brazelton, T. B. "Effects of Prenatal Drugs on the Behavior of the Neonate." *Am. J. Psychiatry* **126**: 1261–1266, 1970.

Brazelton, T. B. "Early Parent–Infant Reciprocity" In: Vaughan, V. C., and Brazelton, T. B. (eds.). *The Family—Can It Be Saved?* Year Book Medical Publishers, Chicago, 1976.

Bronfenbrenner, U. *The Two Worlds of Childhood: USA and USSR*. Russel Sage Foundation, New York, 1970.

Brownmiller, S., *Against Our Will: Men, Women and Rape*. Simon & Schuster, New York, 1975.

Busse, E., and Pfeiffer, E. *Behavior and Adaptation in Late Life*. Little, Brown & Co., Boston, 1969.

Cade, T. (ed.). *The Black Woman: An Anthology*. New American Library, New York, 1970.

Cleaver, E. *Soul on Ice*. Dell-Delta/Ramparts, New York, 1968.

Cooperstock, R. "Psychotropic Drug Use among Women." *Can. Med. Assoc. J.* **115**:760–763, 1976.

Corea, G. *The Hidden Malpractice: How American Medicine Treats Women as Patients and Professionals*. William Morrow & Co., New York, 1977.

De Mause, L. (ed.). *The History of Childhood*. Psychohistory Press, New York, 1974.

Dodson, B. *Liberating Masturbation*. Bodysex Designs, New York, 1974.

Ehrenreich, B., and English, P. *Complaints and Disorders: The Sexual Politics of Sickness*. Feminist Press, Old Westbury, New York, 1973.

Eisenberg, L., "Caring for Children and Working: Dilemmas of Contemporary Womanhood." *Pediatrics* **56**:24–28, 1975.

Fee, E. "Woman and Health Care: A Comparison of Theories." *Int. J. Health Services* **5**:397–415, 1975.

Filene, P. *Him/Her/Self, Sex Roles in Modern America*. Harcourt Brace Jovanovich, New York, 1975.

Freeman, Ellen W. "Influence of Personality Attributes on Abortion Experiences." *Am. J. Orthopsychiatry* **47**(3):503–513, July 1977.

Gil, D. *Violence against Children: Physical Child Abuse in the United States*. Harvard University Press, Cambridge, 1970.

Greenblatt, M., and Schuckit, M. A. *Alcoholism Problems in Women and Children*. Grune & Stratton, New York, 1976.

Hays, H. R. *The Dangerous Sex: The Myth of Feminine Evil*. Putnam Books, New York, 1964.

Hilberman, E. *The Rape Victim*. American Psychiatric Association, Washington, D.C., 1976.

Hite, S. *The Hite Report*. Dell, New York, 1976.

Howell, M. C. "Employed Mothers and Their Families." *Pediatrics* **52**:252–263 and 327–343, 1973.

Kaplan, H. I. *The New Sex Therapy: Active Treatment of Sexual Dysfunctions*. Brunner/Mazel, New York, 1974.

Katchadourian, H. A., and Lunde, D. T. *Fundamentals of Human Sexuality*. Holt, Rinehart & Winston, New York, 1972.

Klaus, M. H., and Kennel, J. H. *Maternal–Infant Bonding.* C. V. Mosby, Saint Louis, 1976.

Kline-Graber, G., and Graber, B. *Woman's Orgasm: A Guide to Sexual Satisfaction.* Bobbs-Merrill, Indianapolis, 1975.

Lee, B. *Bobbi Lee: Indian Rebel: Struggles of a Native Canadian Woman.* LSM Press, Richmond, B. C., 1975.

Lerner, G. (ed.). *Black Women in White America: A Documentary History.* Vintage Books, New York, 1972.

Levine, S. V. "Sexism and Psychiatry." *Am. J. Orthopsychiatry* **44**:327–336, 1974.

Maas, H., and Kuypers, J. *From Thirty to Seventy.* Jossey-Bass, San Francisco, 1974.

Maccoby, E. E., and Jacklin, C. N. *The Psychology of Sex Differences.* Stanford University Press, Stanford, 1974.

Martin, D. *Battered Wives.* Glide Publications, San Francisco, 1976.

Martin, D., and Lyon, P. *Lesbian/Woman.* Glide Publications, San Francisco, 1972.

Mill, J. S. *The Subjection of Women.* M.I.T. Press, 1970. Originally published in London, in 1869, by Longmans, Green, Reader & Dyer.

Mostow, E., and Newberry, P. "Work Role and Depression in Women: A Comparison of Workers and Housewives in Treatment." *Am. J. Orthopsychiatry* **45**:538–548, 1975.

Parlee, M. "Psychological Aspects of Menstruation, Childbirth and Menopause: An Overview with Suggestions for Further Research." Presented at the Conference on New Directions for Research on Women, Madison, Wisconsin, May 31–June 2, 1975.

Pleck, J. H., and Sawyer, J. (eds.). *Men and Masculinity.* Spectrum Books, Englewood Cliffs, New Jersey, 1974.

Rosenhan, D. L. "On Being Sane in Insane Places." *Science* **179**:250–258, 1973.

Rosenthal, R., and Jacobson, L. *Pygmalion in the Classroom, Teacher Expectations and Pupil's Intellectual Endowment.* Holt, Rinehart & Winston, New York, 1968.

Russell, D. E. H., and Van de Ver, N. (eds.). *Crimes against Women.* Les Femmes, Millbrae, California, 1976.

Sidel, R. *Women and Child Care in China.* Penguin Books, Baltimore, 1974.

Smith-Rosenberg, C. "The Hysterical Woman: Sex Roles in Nineteenth Century America." *Social Research* **39**:652–678, 1972.

Tennov, D. *Psychotherapy: The Hazardous Cure.* Abelard-Schuman, New York, 1975.

Whishant, K., and Zegans, L. "A Study of Attitudes Towards Menarche in White Middle-Class American Adolescent Girls." *Am. J. Psychiatry* **132**:809–814, 1975.

Section XX. Psychiatric Research and Evaluation

A. History and Philosophy of Psychiatric Research Design

Major References

Bull, J. P. "The Historical Development of Clinical Therapeutic Trials." *J. Chron. Dis.* **10**:218–248, 1959.

Dreitzel, H. P. *Recent Sociology, No. 2: Patterns of Communicative Behavior.* Macmillan, New York, 1972.

Hamburg, D. (ed.). *Psychiatry vs. a Behavioral Science.* Prentice-Hall, Englewood Cliffs, New Jersey, 1970.

Rosen, G. *Madness in Society.* University of Chicago Press, Chicago, 1968.

Scheff, T. (ed.). *Mental Illness and Social Process.* Harper & Row, New York, 1967.

Wooten, B. *Social Science and Social Pathology.* Allen & Unwin, London, 1959.

B. Models, Statistics, and Computers in Psychiatry

Major References

Dreyfus, H. L. *What Computers Can't Do: A Critique of Artificial Reason.* Harper & Row, New York, 1972.

Feinstein, A. R. *Clinical Judgment*. Williams and Wilkins, Baltimore, 1967.

Harre, R. *The Principles of Scientific Thinking*. University of Chicago Press, Chicago, 1970.

Maxwell, A. E. *Basic Statistics in Behavioral Research*. Gannon, Santa Fe, New Mexico, 1970.

Medawar, P. B. *Induction and Intuition in Scientific Thought*. Methuen, London, 1969.

Nathan, P. E. *Cues, Decisions and Diagnosis*. Academic Press, New York, 1967.

Pearce, K. I. "Computer Simulation as an Aid to the Planning of Psychiatric Services." *Can. Psychiatr. Assoc. J.* **12**:219–221, 1967.

Pearce, K. I. "Towards a Completely Computerized Record System." *Can. Psychiatr. Assoc. J.* **14**: 175–190, 1969.

Roth, M. "The Clinical Interview and Psychiatric Diagnosis: Have They a Future in Psychiatric Practice?" *Compr. Psychiatry* **8**:427–438, 1967.

Siegler, M., and Osmond, H. "Models of Madness." *Br. J. Psychiatry* **112**:1193–1203, 1966.

Wood, G. *Fundamentals of Psychological Research*. 2nd ed. Little, Brown, Boston, 1977.

C. Psychiatric Epidemiology as Human Ecology

Major References

Ehrlich, P. R., and Ehrlich, A. H. *Population Resources, Environment*. Freeman, San Francisco, 1970.

Hill, A. B. "The Environment and Disease: Association or Causation." *Proc. R. Soc. Med.* **58**:295–300, 1965.

Kohn, R. *The Health of the Canadian People*. Royal Commission on Health Services, Queen's Printer, Ottawa, 1967.

LeRiche, W. H., and Milner, J. *Epidemiology as Medical Ecology*. Churchill Livingstone, Edinburgh, 1971.

Lin, T. M., and Slandy, C. C. "The Scope of Epidemiology in Psychiatry." *Public Health Papers*, No. 16. World Health Organization, Geneva, 1962.

Philip, A. E., and McCulloch, J. W. "Use of Social Indices in Psychiatric Epidemiology." *Br. J. Prev. Soc. Med.* **20**:122–126, 1966.

Reid, D. D. "Epidemiological Methods in the Study of Mental Disorders." *Public Health Papers*, No. 2. World Health Organization, Geneva, 1960.

Shepherd, M., and Cooper, B. "Epidemiology and Mental Disorder: A Review." *J. Neurol. Neurosurg. Psychiatry* **27**:277–290, 1964.

Thurlow, M. A. "General Susceptibility to Illness: A Selective Review." *Can. Med. Assoc. J.* **97**:1397–1404, 1967.

D. Evaluation of Psychiatric Treatment, Treatment Programs, and Training

Major References

Cooper, D. *Psychiatry and Anti-Psychiatry*. Tavistock, London, 1967.

Hurst, J. W., and Walker, H. K. (eds.). *The Problem-Oriented System*. Medcom Press, New York, 1972.

Suchman, E. A. *Evaluative Research*. Russell Sage Foundation, New York, 1967.